Warrior
Patient

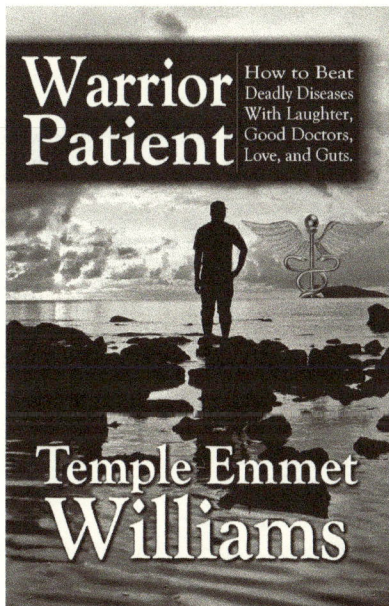

Warrior Patient How to Beat Deadly Diseases With Laughter, Good Doctors, Love, and Guts.

Temple Emmet
Williams

*How to Beat
Deadly Diseases
With Laughter,
Good Doctors,
Love, and Guts.*

Templeworks
Properties, LLC

Published by Templeworks Properties LLC
3755 Mykonos Court, Boca Raton, Florida 33487
(561) 241-6323 Fax: (561) 241-6358

http://www.templeworks.biz
http://www.warriorpatient.com
e-mail: temple@warriorpatient.com

Williams, Temple Emmet
Warrior Patient: How to Beat Deadly Diseases With Laughter,
Good Doctors, Love, and Guts.

1. Memoir 2. Autobiography 3. Health and Wellness 4. Cancer

ISBN-13: : 978-0-9968-9207-0
Library of Congress Control Number: 2015903455

Dedication

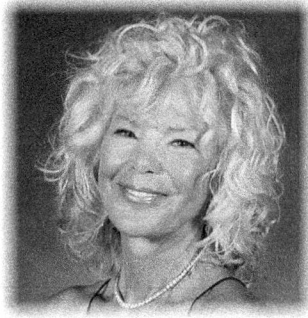

To Kerstin (Kickan) Williams,
who has been saving my life
since the first day we met. in 1971

Books by Temple Emmet Williams

Fiction: Wrinkled Heartbeats
Poison Heartbeats
African Heartbeats
Non-Fiction: Warrior Patient
Warrior Patient Heartbeats

A Note About the Cover

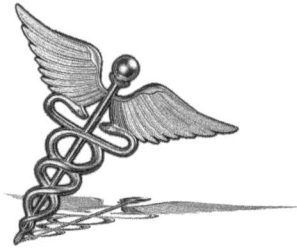

On the cover, a patient stands on rocks looking at a caduceus rising out of an ocean. It's an allegory of hope and a totally, utterly MISLEADING one. The symbolic staff, with two entwined snakes and two wings at the top, is often used by medical practitioners, and yet it has absolutely nothing to do with the practice of Medicine. It is a mistake, particularly prevalent in the United States.

The U.S. Army Medical Corps adopted the caduceus in a patch for their uniforms in 1902. They should have used the Rod of Asclepius, which is the proper symbol of medicine, similar, but quite different. The Rod of Asclepius shows a single serpent wrapped around a rod, no wings in sight. The Greek God Asclepius, who was associated with healing and medicine, wielded his rod to help the sick and those who cared for them.

The addition of two wings and a second serpent proved irresistible to modern medicine.

The caduceus is a powerful symbol of commerce. It represents trade, eloquence, trickery, and negotiation, but never medicine.

On the book's front cover, the patient sees the rising wings and serpents as a sign of hope. By the end of the book, however, he sees it for what it truly represents. Because he does, he survives the most exceptional medical system that our civilization has ever known.

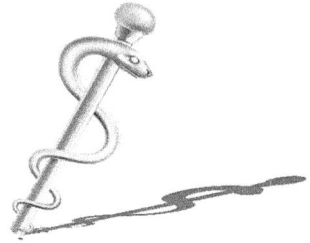

Table of Contents

Chapter 1

The Fall

"All I could think about was sex," your dinner partner tells you. She ...."

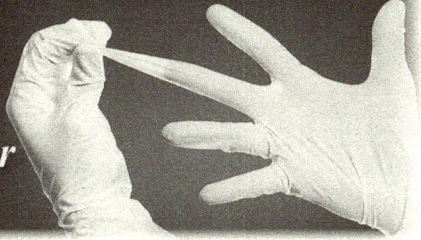

The tennis pro, Gary Kesl, stands outside a white stucco clubhouse. He pulls out his cell phone. He watches the doubles match on Court Three, where aging tennis members suddenly circle a fallen player.

Their voices slice through the autumn heat of Boca Raton, Florida.

"Stay on the ground!"

"Don't move!"

"Are you all right?"

Kids never hear this when they fall on a clay tennis court. They bounce up, embarrassed, and their next shot has extra juice on it. Old guys stay down.

"I'm fine," you tell your tennis buddies. You give them thumbs up, struggle to your feet. You do not know that your journey from medical dope to healthy hope has just begun.

It will include cancer, kidney failure, dialysis, deadly infections, partial blindness, shingles, large open wounds, a hernia, and a little amputation. There will be some brilliant doctors, an exceptional one, one terrible one (who goes to jail), a handful of excellent surgeons, and good and bad nurses. You'll meet a bunch of technicians (one of whom comes close to killing you), and compassionate and careless caregivers. Your blessings include a wife who saves your life, more friends than you knew you had, and lessons in survival that change your life, for better rather than worse.

You still don't remember who won the point of the game or the match when you trip and kiss the clay. Your seemingly harmless fall gives you a back twinge for a few days. A year later, doctors find a hematoma in that area, a blood leak into muscle, with nowhere to go. Your body surrounds it with an envelope, isolates it like water in a balloon. An excellent immune system does this. Life-threatening infection appears at the base of the hematoma. It tries to overpower your reliable immune system.

On the day of the tennis court stumble, you repeat: "I'm fine." Gary Kesl, who played doubles at Wimbledon and coached a lot of world-class tennis stars, pockets his cell phone. He'll put some extra clay on Court 3 and have his assistant work it into the lines later.

Between games, a quick calendar check on your cell phone reminds you that you have an appointment with your primary doctor the next day.

"Can't play tomorrow, guys."

"You hurting?"

"I'm fine. I'm good. Annual check-up. Time for the once-a-year snap of a rubber glove." This reference to getting what doctors call a DRE (digital rectal exam) gets a nervous laugh from all the men. Two of them are prostate cancer survivors.

You step back onto the tennis court, bouncing a little to prove you're okay.

"Serve 'em up," you say. You stretch, lean down and touch the ground without bending your knees. Well, maybe a little. Your partner, Lee Gelfond, watches you. "I'm fine," you say to yourself, as well as to him. "I swear, I'm fine."

"Don't overdo it." He says this often.

That evening, you have a conversation at a dinner party that you repeat to your primary doctor the following day. You do not understand its significance at the time.

"All I could think about was sex," your dinner partner tells you. She is a cute redhead, with a trace of freckles scattered in a tight face. Your wife of 39 years smiles at you from the other side of the table. She can hear a pin drop in a crowded room. Your wife is a beautiful woman. Swedish. An athlete. With a heart that weeps if a tiny frog drowns in your swimming pool. You wake up every morning, thinking you might be the luckiest guy on earth.

You believe it.

You arch your eyebrows at your dinner partner and wonder what she would look like with duct tape over her mouth. She continues:

"It was the only way I could compete with the male traders."

She is talking about testosterone treatments she takes when she is a 32-year-old floor trader at the Chicago Mercantile Exchange. She trades better, matches the aggressive behavior of the men around her, takes uncommon and uncomfortable risks.

She also grows facial hair. You detect no mustache or sideburns, just faded freckles and slight smile lines.

"But it was the sex thing that bothered me the most," she adds. "All I could think about was sex." She stabs some steak on her plate. "I feel sorry for men."

Tough conversation. Tough lady. "Yes," you reply. "Shaving is no fun." You laugh. Your wife giggles on the other side of the table. She must have thought of something funny.

You tell this story to Doctor Efrosini "Susan" Barish, your primary physician, during your annual check-up at Personal Physicians Associates. She's a tall, slender woman with a natural smile, dark-haired, with slightly olive skin from her Greek heritage spread across sharp, attractive features.

You often talk about her daredevil son's ventures around the world. She worries about him with pride.

Doctor Barish smiles at your testosterone story, snapping on her rubber gloves.

"Bend over."

Once again, you expect to have a beautiful, small prostate.

"Have you been taking any testosterone treatments?" she asks. You assume she is continuing the conversation.

"No."

As you pull up your pants and tighten your belt, she looks at the latest lab tests you have taken just before your annual check-up. Her eyebrows move up, painting wrinkles on her forehead, and you feel your forehead mimic this. Something is not right.

"Do you sleep through the night without going to the bathroom?" She's serious.

"No," you admit. "I usually make one or two pit stops." It seems pretty reasonable to you.

She keeps scanning the lab test. "My tennis and golf buddies say I go a lot more often when we're playing nowadays," you add.

It comes as an afterthought. It never has much meaning until right now since you consider yourself pretty healthy, active.

"Your PSA has moved up from 1.2 to 4.2 in the last year," Doctor Barish tells you. "I think we need a biopsy of your prostate."

"What's a PSA?" you ask.

"It's a marker," she explains. "It helps detect possible problems with the prostate."

The prostate-specific antigen (PSA) test measures an enzyme in the blood. The epithelial cells of the prostate produce the protein that causes elevated levels of PSA, which point to prostate problems, including cancer.

Way back in 1986, the Food and Drug Administration (FDA) approved the PSA blood test as a means of determining the effectiveness of prostate cancer treatments.

Today, PSA levels, expressed as nanograms per milliliter, act as an early warning tool for men with prostate cancer.

"What happened to my nice, small prostate?" you ask Doctor Barish. You suddenly realize she has not looked at your latest lab tests before the snapping of the rubber glove for the digital rectal exam. She is seeing the numbers, registering them for the first time.

"Your nice, small prostate is a lot larger than it was a year ago," she tells you. The examination room remains quiet for a moment.

"Well, it's time it grew up," you joke. The doctor does not smile, but she repeats: "We need a biopsy of your prostate."

Most men with an elevated PSA do not have prostate cancer. More likely, they suffer from benign prostate enlargement or inflammation. But for older men, a group in which you qualify, levels above 3 to 4 ng/mL usually indicate the need for a biopsy. Every year, doctors perform about a million prostate biopsies in America.

A third of them point to cancer.

Doctor Susan Barish gives you a urologist's name: Doctor Emanuel Gottenger, Advanced Urology of South Florida. He will perform the biopsy. You need to make an appointment as soon as possible. You leave, convinced it would amount to nothing. Still, you may as well make the appointment. You consider not doing so.

Primary physicians are the gatekeepers of America's health care system. Except for emergencies, you have a hard time playing with doctors or hospitals or nurses or specialists or technicians without their approval. Depending on your medical coverage, you may or may not be able to choose your specialists. Once you are in a hospital, it's tough to get out without the discharge authority from your primary physician.

According to the American Academy of Family Physicians, demand for primary doctors has jumped dramatically. The Academy says that growth in population, aging, and increased coverage will require over 50,000 new primary physicians by the year 2025.

Being a gatekeeper does not pay as well as being a specialist. Because of this, many primary doctors are specialists, too.

The Association of Medical Colleges puts primary care physicians in the penalty box right from the start. High student loans and low pay during residency do not always attract the best and the brightest.

If you are not near the top of your class at medical school, becoming a primary doctor could well be the avenue of least resistance to a successful future.

For many doctors, but especially for primary physicians, referrals are a business, not a filter for quality care. Nevertheless, many patients assume their primary physician has prescribed the best solution, not the easiest or most profitable one.

Patients can pay a terrible price for this.

Consider this scenario (it happens a few months later, but it's a perfect example here of critical, dangerous information).

The phone rings. You hear tears, crying, fear. "I have ovarian cancer," your wife weeps. Words tumble through the phone; each word bruises the next with increasing pain.

"The nurse says she is so sorry she's so sad it's a huge mass according to the doctor, and oh, the nurse looks so scared oh God what am I going to do they can't even see my ovary the mass is so big."

Her words slip into short breaths, a hollow sound, but easily heard.

You and your wife have been together for a long time (48 years during this 2020 revision).

Kerstin is a tough, Swedish-born American, who has run large organizations, started chambers of commerce, run her businesses on her own. She is in tremendous physical and mental shape.

"Are they certain it's ovarian cancer?" You want to climb through the phone. Hold her. Protect her.

"They can see the mass on the ultrasound they just did," she sobs, but a little calmer now. "It's huge. It scared the nurse. You could see it in her face. They can't even see the ovary."

According to the nurse, there is a test they still have to do, which they call a CA-125. It will confirm cancer.

Kerstin returns home to wait for the results. The nurse promises to call as soon as they know anything.

"I know it's bad," Kerstin tells you. "I thought the nurse was going to cry when she talked to me."

Nothing happens for several days, although you both decide a second opinion makes sense. Kerstin asks her primary physician, also Doctor Susan Barish, for another referral.

Before she visits the second ObGyn, Kerstin calls the first referral and asks to speak to the doctor.

She feels as if she is dialing for a firing squad. It is one of the most challenging calls she ever makes.

The nurse comes on the line after a long wait and says: "It was nothing — just a fibroid. The CA-125 is negative. You have nothing to worry about, Kerstin. The doctor says you should NOT have it removed because surgery can always lead to complications."

"It was nothing?" Kerstin whispers into the phone. "Why didn't you call?"

The nurse says nothing. After a while, Kerstin asks if she's still on the line. "I did call," she finally says. "I left a message."

You are a financial trader and a real estate broker. Every call made to your home gets digitally recorded, especially if you are not available. The nurse never called.

In her relief over the negative test for ovarian cancer, Kerstin lets the insult of frightening, careless communication wash away. The aftertaste of misused authority lingers, however, even today. It remains challenging to understand, troubling, and shockingly familiar.

Kerstin decides to continue with the second opinion. The next ObGyn works out of an office that looks like it has not changed in 50 years.

Old furniture displays tattered magazines in poor lighting. It feels tired, tarnished. The doctor and his nurse agree that Kerstin has a fibroid mass.

"We can remove that right away," the doctor says. His assistants start scheduling an operation for Kerstin. Which hospital does she want to use? The Boca Raton Regional? The Delray Medical Center? The doctor has no preference. Things are starting to move very fast.

They shove permissions and authorizations in front of Kerstin. They ask for signatures.

"NO," stops everything. "No!"

Kerstin walks out, comes home, unwilling to fall into the trap of a thoughtless system that views patients as opportunistic revenue streams. She changes her primary physician.

In the end, Kerstin has a non-invasive, outpatient hysterectomy. Her doctor removes the fibroid mass. It is benign. The surgeon is the newly-appointed head of the Cleveland Clinic in West Palm Beach.

Kerstin spends a lot of time identifying the right doctor and approach, using cyberspace and testimonials and success rates as her guide. The operation is simple, successful, and her life returns to normal within days. From start to finish, Kerstin's journey from "You have ovarian cancer" to becoming a successful Warrior Patient lasts less than two months. Your journey takes much longer, over three years.

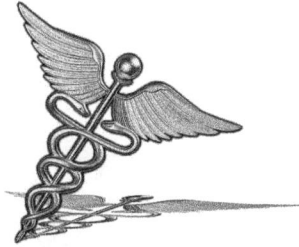

<u>Warrior Patient Rule 1</u>: Choose to live. Take personal responsibility for getting better. It is not your doctor's job. It is not God's job. It is your job. God and your doctors might help. And they might not.

Chapter 2

You Have Cancer

"He's being treated up in Orlando." Kerstin says. "By a robot."

"We're going to give you a local anesthetic to numb things up, and then the doctor will perform the biopsy," the nurse says. She shows you into a small room at the urologist's office, with an examination table and a chair and some medical equipment that means nothing to you.

"We take pictures as we do it," she says.

"I'm sorry about the cat pee," you answer, kicking off your shoes and sliding them quickly under the chair.

"I beg your pardon?" the nurse asks.

"One of our cats took a pee in my loafers, and they stink a little," you say. "I never smelled it until I was in the car on my way here. Guess I should have gone back and changed my shoes, but I didn't want to be late for my 45-minute layover in your waiting room." Her eyes get a little skinny. You consider apologizing for being on time for the appointment.

"I think it was Truffles," you say. "That's the name of the cat."

The nurse says. "First, we take photos, and the doctor takes samples of different areas of your prostate, which we send in for analysis. We'll know next week."

"A feral cat invaded our courtyard; that's what made Truffles do it," you say. "I'm going to have to toss the loafers."

You focus more on the cat's territorial rights and bad manners than on the possibility of prostate cancer. You feel fine. They won't discover anything.

The nurse holds up a black, snake-like ultrasound probe. A biopsy gun gleams at the end of it. It is the gun that will fire a needle through the wall of your rectum.

"The camera," she says, simplifying the device. You suddenly have no concern about the cat or your stinking loafers.

You immediately recognize this ultrasound probe as the spawn of giant pythons invading the Florida Everglades.

"I'll try to focus," you say, adding: "You have a very nice waiting room."

The urologist appears, Doctor Emanuel Gottenger, Advanced Urology of South Florida. He's a stocky guy who probably could shave twice a day. South America gives his voice an unusual cadence, somewhat soothing, but matter-of-fact, professional. You don't expect you'll see very much of him in your life. You are two strangers passing in an examination room that you will never visit again.

Rubber gloves snap. You get numbed with a local anesthetic, and you lay on your side. You are quiet during the 15-minute procedure. The probe emits sound waves that convert different prostate zones into video images. The urologist explains the process while he does it. "You'll hear a clicking sound, and that's the device taking off a thin strip of tissue from one of the sectors the pathologist will analyze. There will be a dozen strips. You shouldn't feel anything."

Click. Pause. Click. Pause. The seventh click gets repeated in the same area, and there's a slight twinge of pain, more of a surprise than anything else. Then you're done.

You ask to see his handiwork. He shows you a dozen little vials, each with a tiny worm-like strip of pink tissue in it.

"See you next week," Doctor Gottenger says. "They'll set up an appointment on the way out. Why does it smell like cat pee in here?" The nurse points at your offending loafers under the chair. You start to explain, but the urologist is already out the door.

"Turn right and make an appointment at the desk," the nurse tells you, trailing after him.

"See you next week," you tell nobody, as you finish dressing to leave.

You give little thought to the biopsy during the next seven days. You play tennis, golf, go biking and swimming, and build a computer from scratch. You recognize the last as a distraction. You understand and enjoy machines, having spent several years as the leading contractor for creative services at IBM's multimedia laboratory in Palisades, NY. In youth, you messed with cars. Now you buy motherboards and daughterboards and processors and disc drives and build a super-fast black box that welcomes every corner of the world into your home through the internet.

During the week, tissue samples from your biopsy slip under the microscope of a pathologist. He or she records a description of each and the area of the prostate from which it came. The specifications define the cell samples as normal (benign), suspicious (atypical), or malignant (cancer).

Malignant cells receive a grade based on their appearance. The grading determines how aggressive cancer has become. Low-grade cancer cells appear close to normal. Intermediate-grade cells have lost many of their features. They look sloppy and disorganized. High-grade cancer cells appear distorted to the point where they bear little resemblance to healthy cells.

Pathologists require at least four years of residency training beyond their four years of medical school. Many have sub-specialty training in disciplines such as urology. The pathologist examines the core specimens, looking for something called a Gleason Score, which currently benchmarks whether or not you have cancer and its degree of severity.

The most normal looking malignant cells have a Gleason pattern of "1." The worst looking cells rate a "5." This numbers game adds up the primary and secondary model within a malignant tumor to arrive at the Gleason score. The primary grade carries more weight than the second one in determining the aggressiveness of cancer. If the primary degree is "3," and the second grade is "4," the Gleason score would be "7" or "3+4." However, if the primary category is "4" and the second grade is "3," the Gleason score would be "4+3," also "7," but more aggressive, more dangerous because the primary category registered a "4."

Of course, you do not understand any of this at the time. It is not essential since there is nothing wrong with you.

A week later, you return to the urologist's office for a meeting the physician has every year with dozens of patients. Doctor Gottenger is about to admit it is all a false alarm. Maybe you have a touch of Prostatitis.

One of your tennis buddies suggests that it might be your problem.

"Naturally," the Doctor Gottenger says, "you have cancer."

You feel nothing at first. No shock. A little curiosity at the use of the word "naturally" perhaps. Then you feel your mind shift. You watch the doctor talking, but very little of what he says gets inside your head. The sound is off. Lips move, but you hear nothing.

"Excuse me, Doc," you say. "Can we start over? I have cancer?"

Doctor Gottenger rewinds the tape. "Your Gleason score is four plus three," he says. "You have a lot of alternatives."

"But, I have cancer."

He looks up from the pathology report spread in front of him.

"Yes," he answers, "you have cancer. But if you're going to get cancer, this is probably the one you want. You have a lot of alternatives, a lot of different treatments, ranging from doing nothing and monitoring it very carefully to having a doctor take out your prostate completely with radical prostatectomy."

"My mother had cancer," you say. The statement comes out of nowhere. "She lived to ninety-four. My grandmother lived to one hundred and four."

Doctor Gottenger leans back in his chair and watches you, and you quickly realize he is doing this. Somehow, you have arrived at a dangerous point.

You take a deep breath as if you have just finished a grueling race. You fall back into the moment.

"Alternatives," you say. You and the doctor discuss them, and you have a lot of alternatives. You have cancer.

When you get home, you hug Kerstin. "Great news," you say. "Doctor Gottenger says as long as I have cancer, this is the one I want." It takes a moment for this to register. Her initial smile flattens out.

The edges of her mouth turn lower.

"You have cancer." It's a statement, not a question. You nod. She sits down. You talk.

Prostate cancer is the second most common cancer in American males (trailing skin cancer). Over a quarter of a million men get it every year, according to the American Cancer Society. Over 12% of them will eventually drop dead from it, but that number steadily slides lower because of new and improved treatment options.

Lung cancer pushes more American men into the grave, but prostate cancer has an excellent lock on second place. It was before Covid-19 got in the race.

"I want cancer out of my body," you tell Kerstin. She agrees. The shadow of cancer scares both of us. You do not realize at this stage that virtually all of the men diagnosed with prostate cancer remain alive five years later. Ten years later, 98% of them relax on the right side of the grass. Even after 15 years, 93% of them sit up in the morning without hitting their head on wood.

Death stalks men with prostate cancer, but it does not wear running shoes.

"I want cancer out of my body ... now," you repeat. You look at Kerstin and say: "When my mother had breast cancer, she immediately had a double mastectomy." Kerstin knows this.

"We are the children of our mother," you say softly. You are not blaming cancer on your mother, merely explaining the path you will take, preordained, hereditary. You are, at this stage, a medical dope.

Your grandfather's brother, Robert Emmet, served as an Admiral in the Navy. When you are a small child, Uncle Bob tells you: "In life, you will make good decisions, you will make bad decisions. But you must make decisions. If they are the wrong ones, you will know. You will lose." Your mother's decision to knife cancer out of her body works out well. She lives another 45 years, all but the last two with youthful energy and laughter.

When you have cancer, most of your friends offer well-meaning advice. When you have prostate cancer, a surprising number of them admit they were in line in front of you. Welcome aboard.

Everyone knows the perfect doctor (theirs), the correct procedure (the one they had), and they all have incontrovertible proof that they are right (they're still breathing).

"Orvar has prostate cancer," Kerstin says. He is an extraordinary Swedish friend, generous and genuine, a great businessman with an equally tough wife. She manages to contain his appetites for life as if she were a ringmaster in a lion's cage. You admire them both. "He's in a hospital up in Orlando," Kerstin says. "With a robot." You laugh. You know about robotic surgery, but it is just a modern curiosity until now.

You have a good friend, a tennis partner you play doubles with when your team wins the Palm Beach County championship in your division. You never lose during the season. Richard Yules is a general in the Air Force and a medical doctor, an actual general doctor you joke (probably too often).

Dick is fierce and funny and always a general, even when his uniform hangs, retired, in the closet. They diagnose his prostate cancer earlier than yours. He has a simple answer. Get it out. Get rid of it. Your cancer attitude will rhyme with his.

Dick knows some of the best doctors in the world, and he uses his knowledge of the system to free himself of cancer within weeks of the diagnosis. He makes the decision. He lives by it, and perhaps because of it.

But there are many alternatives to "get cancer out of me, get rid of it." They fall into four general categories: active surveillance, radiation, hormone therapy, and surgery.

According to Johns Hopkins Hospital, considered a Mecca of medicine, no "best" choice of treatment exists.

Too many variables, such as age, health, personal preference, and a man's prostate risk level, make it hard to nail down an overall treatment winner.

But if you expect to live another decade or more, then you need some approach because cancer has an 80% chance of getting worse.

Johns Hopkins has been ranked the No.1 hospital in America by U.S. News & World Report for 21 years in a row. Their white papers on prostate disorders have a reputation that approaches biblical proportions.

The do-nothing approach of active surveillance makes sense for older people with prostate cancer, especially if it's low risk. The trauma of surgery or radiation, or complications from any treatment, can kill them. "The operation was a great success," the doctor says. "But the patient died."

Radiation therapy can leave a patient cancer-free for ten years or longer. Combined with hormonal treatments, skilled radiation oncologists (cancer doctors) have many choices. With three-dimensional imaging, they can destroy cancer with greater accuracy and higher doses. That means fewer or reduced side effects (blood in the urine, incontinence, ulcers in the intestines, erectile dysfunction, bladder problems, and anal cancer).

With another type of radiation therapy, Brachytherapy, oncologists implant up to a hundred radioactive metal pellets in the prostate. The pellets emit cancer-destroying radiation for several months. After they are "spent," they remain in the prostate, harmless. It's called permanent low-dose-rate Brachytherapy. Although the dosage rate dies after a few months, the seeds hang around forever.

A new approach implants high-dose pellets for a day or two. Then they remove them. Research suggests that this new approach does not improve the outcome, but patients have fewer problems with urinary frequency, incontinence, blood in the urine, and rectal pain.

Another approach is cryotherapy, which kills the cancer cells by freezing them. It's quite a complicated treatment.

Ice balls inserted into the prostate through thin needles freeze the entire organ. A warm saline solution protects other areas to prevent them from freezing.

They use this procedure when radiation therapy fails to halt prostate cancer.

Hormonal treatment can fight prostate cancer, but it cannot cure it. The cancer cells learn how to work around the hormone treatment by producing the hormones that they need. Cancer keeps growing, destroying healthy cells and organs. Still, hormone therapy prolongs the life of men with severe prostate cancer.

The side effects, however, remain exceedingly tough. They almost certainly include erectile dysfunction (hormonal treatment aims to reduce the male sex hormone testosterone).

Patients suffer the loss of libido (sex drive), breast enlargement, weight gain, muscle loss, fatigue, hot flashes, and osteoporosis (bone loss). Some think the cure may be worse than the disease.

Chemotherapy can help relieve pain and the symptoms of very advanced prostate cancer. Doctors use it when hormonal therapy fails. The survival advantage, however, remains a matter of months, not years. Some new drugs and drug combinations offer promise. But this approach still resembles guinea pig alley, which often, and rightly, looks like an open road to men facing immediate death.

Surgery can cure prostate cancer, get rid of it altogether, and put a "cancer-free" stamp of approval on a man's life. It only works if cancer has not spread beyond the prostate.

A friend with cancer tells you that there only two reasonable choices on the road to success: a skilled surgeon or an experienced surgeon using a robot.

You have already decided on a radical prostatectomy.

Yank it out.

Get rid of cancer.

You will follow in the footsteps of your Swedish friend Orvar.

You will sign up for surgery at the Global Robotics Institute in Orlando, Florida.

The leading robotic prostate surgeon in the world, Doctor Vipul Patel, will set you free.

Because you are a medical dope at this stage, you do not realize that Johns Hopkins, the No.1 hospital in America for 21 years in a row, thinks that you are making a pretty bad decision.

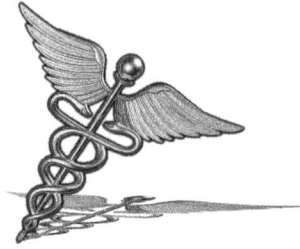

<u>Warrior Patient Rule 2</u>: The internet unlocks everything you need to know about doctors, hospitals, procedures, and treatments. A mouse, a click, or finger swipe will put you on the right road to solving your medical problems.

Chapter 3

The Catheter Wars

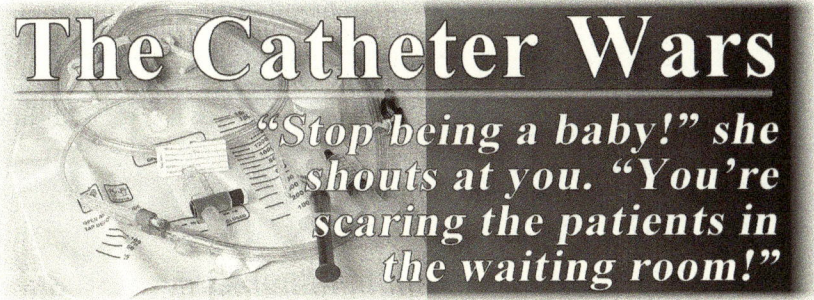

"Stop being a baby!" she shouts at you. "You're scaring the patients in the waiting room!"

Doctor Ivan Coronado, your wife's cardiologist, asks: "Why do you think Doctor Patel needs so many tests done before the surgery?" He's taking an EKG and giving you a stress test before your acceptance as a patient at the Global Robotics Institute in Florida. Diodes cover your body, and you continue panting from the stress test.

"Patel's covering his ass," you answer.

Doctor Coronado's mouth makes an "O" and duplicates the sound: "Oh." He looks down at a printout and says: "Not holding back on opinions, are we?"

The test is one of many medical hoops you must jump through before Doctor Vipul Patel, and his robot will gently remove your troubled prostate. The barrage of requirements to get through the doors of the Global Robotics Institute seems overwhelming when you sign up for your radical prostatectomy shortly after the biopsy. It is three months before the scheduled surgery can occur. Doctor Patel is an extremely busy guy.

Shortly before the procedure, you send an e-mail to your good friend and actual General Doctor, Richard Yules."I'm two weeks away from rip and strip in Orlando," you write. "Interesting journey. All the qualities of life. Pain. Agony. Catheters. Character-building stuff."

You tell him: "I have seen the best and worst of a system that has turned doctoring from an act of benevolent courage into a system of covering your ass. For Heaven's sake, I want them to cover MY ass, not theirs."

You end the e-mail with flippant hope: "... I have been stress-tested, X-Rayed, ultra-sounded (not sure that's a word), and declared suitable for drawing and quartering in Orlando under the auspices of Doctor Patel and his robot. He's done over 5000 robotic procedures, and some of them are still upright, so I am comfortable with whatever happens."

But you are far from comfortable getting to this point because there are some unexpected, character-building events in the months leading up to the robotic operation.

Right after the biopsy, everything appears normal. Doctor Gottenger gives you a four-day supply of Ciprofloxacin, a powerful antibiotic. It seems to work, but only for a few days. After a week has passed, something is wrong. You are in a great deal of pain, and you have a difficult time going to the bathroom. Your urine becomes dark instead of pale yellow.

In the examination room, Doctor Gottenger asks nobody in particular: "I wonder why you're so infected?" You guess that it explains your dark urine.

You think it is an excellent question. It deserves an answer.

Instead, Doctor Gottenger prescribes another antibiotic for ten days. Perhaps he feels you are on the way to Florida Hospital in

Orlando, and the radical prostatectomy will solve all your problems. That's the only rationalization you have for his lack of an answer to his question. The new antibiotic pills do not do much, but three days after the final dose, things look like they might be getting better, at least for a while.

You arrive at the point at which you suffer from being a medical dope. You do not demand any answers. You only request treatment. You do not know how to listen to your body, which is an acquired ability; it does not just happen. As your capacity to listen gets better, it tells you what is good to eat and what is not. Or whether or not a doctor's advice is helping you. Or whether the pain in your stomach is gas or something more serious. Your body speaks to you, but you must know how to listen. Women are better at this than men.

So at this stage, you are not a Warrior Patient. You trust a doctor who listens to your body. He knows you have an infection. He sees it. But rather than discover its source, he hands you off to a procedure that he assumes will take care of it.

It is easy to be stupid in an age of miracles. It can also be deadly.

Medicine is not magic, and doctors are not magicians. But in every culture, the medicine man assumes the mantle of an all-powerful demigod. As patients, we willingly raise them to that level with acclaim and applause. Bad doctors continue to bury their mistakes, and nobody hands out a Nobel Prize to patients who survive bad doctors.

Those who do not believe in the religion of modern medicine become easy prey for quacks and mystical cures. You understand that modern medicine has a leg up on twigs, bark, and grazing on lemongrass with flowers in your hair. You recognized the importance of traditional medicine and caregivers. You know, of course, that nobody gets out of life alive.

Had you been a Warrior Patient at this point, you would realize that the biopsy has somehow opened a gate to infection. It might not be the cause of the infection, but it certainly throws out a welcome mat for the inflammation of your prostate. Doctor Gottenger might dispute this, but at the very least, a good doctor should examine your problem beyond "I wonder why you're so infected?"

You have already had a full-body scan and ultrasound examination of your pelvic region in preparation for robotic surgery. Those examinations reveal no problems. They cannot also detect infections.

A month after the biopsy, you are "good to go" for the radical prostatectomy with Doctor Patel at Florida Hospital in Orlando. You have taken all the preliminary tests to qualify for Doctor Patel's robotic surgery.

You are also in the Emergency Room at the Delray Medical Center, bent over with acute, breath-taking pain.

"Where does it hurt?" the emergency room receptionist asks. You answer in short sentences.

"Can't pee. Gonna explode."

You push your Medicare card across the shelving that separates the receptionist from the patients. You bend in half. That's how you walk through the emergency door. Kerstin drops you off at the entrance and parks the car.

"Bladder will burst. Hard to talk."

The receptionist asks if you have been a patient at the Delray Hospital before.

You nod frantically, bending over at a 45-degree angle.

She types information from your Medicare card into her computer, and she asks you for your birth date.

She discovers that you broke your collarbone in a bike accident a few years earlier. She's typing with two fingers, and you think she needs to take a typing class. She pushes the card back to you.

"Have a seat," she smiles. "Someone will be right with you."

"Gonna die," you answer.

You shuffle over to a nearby plastic chair. You grip the back of it, but do not sit. There are only three other people in the emergency intake area. They seem far too relaxed.

Kerstin joins you. She asks what's happening, and you grunt. She walks up to the receptionist and says something. She returns and says: "They're going to take you right away."

"Right away" has already passed. "If I was bleeding badly, I might get faster treatment," you tell Kerstin. "If you have a knife, stab me in the back. It'll work. I promise."

She humors me.

She makes a big deal out of looking in her purse for something long and sharp. She has left her Jim Bowie hunting knife at home. The orderlies come to get you reasonably quickly, but seconds seem to stretch into minutes, and minutes feel like hours.

The hospital staff puts you in a wheelchair and pushes you through the double doors to the emergency room, with Kerstin at your side. You are about to be saved.

But first, they need to take your blood pressure and ask you a few questions. Triage, the priority of treatment based on the severity of a patient's condition, does not favor a bellyache that stumbles into the emergency room on bent knees. "From now on," you tell Kerstin, "we dial nine-one-one."

You manage to tell them that you have prostate cancer, scheduled for radical prostatectomy, in March, robotic, Barish primary, Gottenger urologist, Holy Mother of God, how do women have babies?

"Have you ever had a catheter?" the emergency doctor asks you.

"No!" you bark. Kerstin confirms this, but with more nobility. You apologize. Don't want to give anyone the wrong impression. "I'd love one," you say. "Now."

A nurse inserts a tube through your penis and into your bladder. Almost immediately, you think this is the kindest, most beautiful thing anyone has ever done for you. The relief is spectacular. The nurse and doctor walk out of the triage cubicle, and you fall sound asleep, holding Kerstin's hand. They wake you and, after about thirty minutes and some paperwork, you return home. You feel as if you have run ten miles, but you have no pain, just soreness.

In your driveway, you pull up your pant leg and show Kerstin the bottom of the plastic drainage bag, held on your leg with elastic bands.

"I have been bagged and tagged," you say. Inside, you discuss the event. You already have a previously arranged appointment with Doctor Gottenger the next day.

"Hey," you tell Kerstin, "my timing is perfect, huh?"

She looks at you sideways. She will not humor a medical dope.

"The biopsy gave you an infection," she says. "I don't like Doctor Gottenger."

"He's not a bad guy," you say.

"I hate him," she says.

"You don't hate anybody," you point out. "That's my job." Whenever you say you hate somebody, Kerstin warns you that you should not hate anybody or anything.

Life is all about love.

"I don't hate him," she says. "You know what I mean." And you guess you do.

The next day, you arrive at Doctor Gottenger's office five minutes early and have another long layover before an assistant finally calls your name and invites you through the door to the inner sanctum of urology.

You tell the emergency room story to Doctor Gottenger with as much dramatic enthusiasm as you can muster.

"I couldn't pee for almost two days," you tell him. "I have a pretty high pain threshold, but this was unbelievable. I thought I was having a baby." He nods at you.

"It can be excruciating," he admits. They have already taken a sample of your urine and tested it. He decides to keep you catheterized for a week, and then we will all see what happens. "The color of your urine is not too bad," he says. "There is no hematuria."

He looks at your blank stare and says: "That means blood in the urine."

He makes some notes and stands up, saying a nurse will be in to swap out your catheter. "Then make an appointment at the desk, and I will see you in a week."

The back of his white jacket turns left out the door of the examination room.

They replace your brand new catheter with another brand new catheter. The bag is different, but the connections seem the same. You wonder if there's an excellent investment opportunity in catheters. The nurse, named Angel, who swaps the catheters, tells you that it's essential to empty the collection bag two or three times a day.

"How long do you keep using the catheter?" you ask. If these things are good for less than a week, you're going to invest in a catheter company.

Angel is a beautiful girl, with a demeanor as gentle as her voice, as soft as her name. Does it get any better than a dark-haired nurse named Angel? "The tubing needs to be changed once a month," she says. "But I think the doctor will probably remove it next week." She tells you to drink plenty of water. "You don't want to get bladder stones," she says.

"No bladder stones," you repeat. Maybe she'd like to hear the tale of your gallbladder operation thirty years earlier. It's a funny story about a weird hospital roommate who worked in a morgue and wanted to include your removed gallstone in his private collection.

"Make an appointment, and we'll see you in a week," she says, walking out.

Your bladder is a balloon-shaped muscle. It contracts when you need to pee, pushing urine through a man's urethra, the tube that runs through the penis. The plumbing in females covers less distance, but the mechanics are the same. When the bladder muscles flex, the muscles around the escape route relax. Everything operates on automatic.

A urinary catheter (also called a Foley in honor of its designer Frederic Foley, a Boston surgeon in the 1930s) is a thin, flexible hose that snakes into your body. It has a small balloon on the end that enters your bladder. They inflate the balloon with sterile water, locking it into place. They deflate it for removal.

The other end of the catheter connects to a collection pouch. You have daytime and nighttime bags. The daytime bag straps around your leg, and the nighttime bag hangs from the side of your bed.

The biggest problem with catheters has always been bacteria. Urinary tract infection remains the most common type of hospital-acquired infection, according to articles from the

American College of Emergency Physicians and the Journal of Emergency Nursing.

The longer a catheter stays in place, the more likely a patient will get a urinary tract or bladder infection. Any sign of redness, swelling, bloody discharge, fever, or lower abdominal pain calls for a quick trip to the emergency room.

You have none of these problems. You pay close attention to personal hygiene, and you love your catheter. A week later, Angel pulls the plug.

Your bladder is ready to fly solo again. It works for a while. Each day, however, it becomes increasingly difficult to take a leak. You struggle through one weekend, but as the next one approaches, you realize you are not going to make it. Dr. Gottenger's office will be closed. It will mean the emergency room again.

Kerstin accompanies you to Doctor Gottenger's office this time. You have squeezed in a late-day appointment. You know your bladder is full, with no relief in sight. Your teeth hurt. Your mind says go, but your body says no. Nothing is working right. You walk up to the reception desk at Advanced Urology of South

Florida and quietly beg receptionist to let you through to the bathroom.

"The Doctor will be with you in a moment, sir," she says.

"NOW," you say, loud enough to draw attention from the patient area. She lets you in, gives you a specimen jar. You go to the bathroom. Close your eyes. Squeeze. Squeeze harder. Red face it.

Not a drop.

Once again, you Angel catheterized you. This time, you are silent, you feel beaten, and you are angry. You look forward to getting to the Global Robotics Institute near Orlando, Florida. You go home and manage to move the surgery date forward a week.

You go for another abdominal scan, and it shows some distention in your bladder, from a circle to an oval.

Several weeks go by, and they try, once again, to remove your catheter. They do it early in the morning. If you can't relieve yourself by around 3:30 pm, you will return to Doctor Gottenger's office and continue catheterization.

By 3 pm, you are in acute pain. It is worse than before. You are having twins. Thirty minutes later, you are having triplets. You shout at Kerstin that you must go to Doctor Gottenger's office immediately. She hurries and is in the process of shutting down her computer when you back out of the drive and head to the urology office on your own. You do not know if you can make it.

You stop at a traffic light on Atlantic Avenue, less than half a mile from the doctor's office. It only takes twenty seconds for the green left-turn arrow to appear, but someone has slowed down the second hand on the traffic coordinator's watch. You try to stand up in the car, your shoulders pressed against the roof, hunched over the steering wheel, moaning. The person in the car next to you has an open mouth staring at you, but she looks away when you grimace at her. You think you might have fouled yourself, but there is no smell. Tears roll down your cheeks.

The light turns, and you race to the doctor's office, strangling the steering wheel.

You park wrongly and stumble into the reception area.

"I need the bathroom, fast!"

"Your name, sir?"

"Goddammit, let me in!" You yank on the door handle that leads to the toilets behind the reception area. You will break the door down if you have to.

"Sir!"

"I am going to crap on your frigging floor!" you say through clenched teeth. You're not confident that you say frigging.

The door clicks, and you are through. You can barely walk, and your cell phone is ringing for the third time. You are on the toilet and can see that you have not fouled yourself. But you cannot pee. You return Kerstin's call, tell her you made it OK and not to worry. You apologize for leaving without her.

Two nurses bring you into an examination room and stretch you out on the paper-covered examination chair. Stretching out your body becomes an excruciating experience. The nurses do not seem very happy with you.

"Jesus, it hurts," you tell the older nurse. Angel is behind her, watching. You bang your head on the back of the examination bench methodically. If you make something else hurt, maybe the excruciating pain in your bladder will go away.

"Stop it," the older nurse orders. You start to groan with pain, which is the worst it has ever been. "Stop it!" she shouts again. You continue to moan and bang your head on the back of the patient's bench. You have no voice, and you can say nothing. Pain fills every fiber of your body — total agony.

The nurse turns and ushers Angel out of the examination room. She slams the door. They have left you alone. Thud. Moan. Thud. Moan. Thud. Moan. You are making a lot of noise. You cannot help it. The only thing that can replace the moan will be a scream. You hold it back. You will not scream. They are torturing you, and you will not yell out.

The door bursts open. "Stop being a baby!" the older nurse shouts at you. "You're scaring the patients in the waiting room!"

You did not know there were patients in the waiting room. You do not even remember stumbling past them.

The nurse jams a catheter into you. She does not do this gently, but the relief is immediate. The pain vanishes, and you close your eyes. Your entire body sags with gratitude.

"Thank you," you say, opening your eyes. The room is empty again, and the door has been closed. You are alone.

You do not see Doctor Gottenger. You dress and walk out to the appointment area, where nobody looks at you. You walk into the waiting room. There are half a dozen people there, and they are all studying their shoes with enormous interest.

"Run," you tell them. "Make a break for it before the nurses get you, too!" Then a genuine laugh escapes from your throat. You shake your head and say, "Sorry."

A few cautious smiles follow you to the exit. At home, you tell Kerstin: "If anyone tries to remove my catheter again, I'll rip off their head and spit down their neck."

You learn this phrase more than fifty years earlier from your Drill Instructor at the Marine Corps boot camp. You are going to get the Dress Blues Award as the top Leatherneck in your barracks. Staff Sergeant Rhyder, your Drill Instructor, finds you dozing behind your bunk the day before you graduate from boot camp at Parris Island, South Carolina. He teaches you the "spitting down your neck" phrase with enormous sincerity and emotion. After the graduation ceremony, you stand in front of him in your Dress Blues and thank him. You are no longer a recruit. You receive a meritorious promotion to Private First Class. He is still your Drill Instructor and will be forever.

After you meet Kerstin over a decade later, she finds your Dress Blues hanging in a closet. She takes off all the brass buttons and turns it into a nice hippie jacket — times change.

"I don't like Doctor Gottenger," Kerstin tells you one more time.

"But you don't hate Doctor Gottenger," you smile, and then you both laugh. It will be over a year and a half before you see Doctor

Gottenger again. Many other doctors play a role in your survival before that reunion occurs. Right now, you are bagged and tagged, and nobody will take your wonderful catheter away from you without risking their life.

The first glimmer of a Warrior Patient has suddenly appeared.

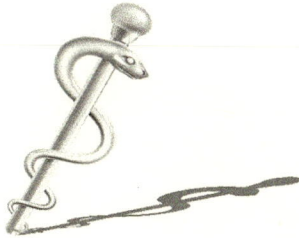

Warrior Patient Rule 3: Do not accept medical abuse from nurses or technicians. Doctors must eliminate any barriers to good health and human kindness in their offices, a clinic, a hospital, or any medical facility. Always.

Chapter 4

Celebration, Florida

"I'm in good hands."
"It's a robot," she says.
"Yeah, but the robot
is in good hands."

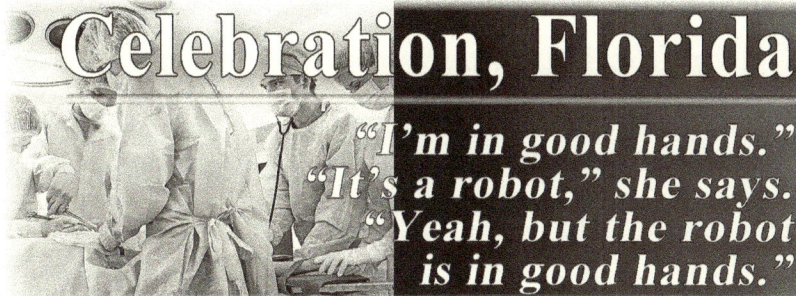

People who live in Boca Raton, where you have lived for several decades, argue over the origin of the city's name. Some say it translates from Spanish as: "Mouth of the Rat"—a rough characterization of an aerial view of its harbor inlet on the Atlantic Ocean. Others suggest a looser translation from older Spanish: "The Bay of the Pirates."

Even today, some search for treasure on its five miles of sun-swept beaches (just don't get caught digging holes in the sand; only sea turtles can do that). Boca Raton lies 35 miles north of Miami's city boundary, and about as many miles south of Palm Beach.

Your robotic prostatectomy is at the Global Robotics Institute of Florida Hospital in Celebration, bordering Orlando. The Disney Development Company invented the town of Celebration, dumping around two and a half billion dollars into 10.7 square miles, almost none of which is water (no swampland for Mickey Mouse).

Less than 8,000 people live in Celebration. The Urban Land Institute named it the "New Community of the Year" shortly after the start of this century.

It's a three to four-hour drive north from Boca on the Florida Turnpike, closer to three if Kerstin's foot is on the pedal, which it is. "I like the name Celebration," she says.

You finish her thought: "I hope it lives up to its name."

The Rules of Engagement for your operation are simple. No food. No water. Nothing remains between your mouth and your butt. A drink that you take the night before guarantees you're running on empty. The concoction tastes like flat, sour cherry soda pop.

"We'd better stop for gas," Kerstin says 100 miles north of Boca.

"I don't have any," you answer. "I'm clean as a whistle." You laugh, in high spirits, heading for the finish line.

You stop to get gas. Your catheter bag still registers empty.

Shortly before the Global Positioning System (GPS) guides you into Kissimmee, which is geographically synonymous with Celebration, you stop and get a Popsicle. The Rules of Engagement permit this.

You have not had a Popsicle in 20 years.

You forget how good they are.

As Kerstin drives the car into what is officially called Florida Hospital Celebration Health, you say, "It does look like a resort, not a hospital."

Manicured landscapes separate large, human-made lakes.

Only the vast "Patient Parking" area suggests it's not all laughter and fun in the sun.

You have a brochure in your hand, and you glance at it.

"A one hundred and twelve-bed, state-of-the-art facility dedicated to beating the crap out of twenty-first-century diseases."

"It does not say that," Kerstin tells me.

"I'm translating from the English," you tell your Swedish wife.

High spirits. And it does look like a resort: lots of glass and Florida pastel colors. Through some of the glass, you see an Olympic-size swimming pool and a well-machined workout area. Kerstin will receive free access to this while Doctor Patel and his robot take care of my prostate problem.

Kerstin has forgotten her bathing suit.

Kerstin will go shopping.

They built Florida Hospital Celebration in 1997 as one of the cornerstones of Disney's planned community. A Mediterranean resort-style facility, it has a 60,000 square foot fitness center and day SPA, concierge service, and a bistro with a head chef who used to work at the Four Seasons. No kidding.

You walk into the spacious facility with high vaulted ceilings. You are reminded of your first trip to New York City as a kid, gawking at things like a dumbfounded tourist.

"These floors look very clean," you say. "I bet you could lick them."

She narrows her eyes, points her finger at you, and says: "Don't!"

She thinks she knows you so well. She thinks you're a child, immature. You don't even think this color of floor tastes that good. High spirits make you smile at her.

A concierge greets you, and she escorts you to the surgery area. She walks you through the process. Not the procedure, just the process. Anesthesia. Surgery. Recovery. Private room. Discharge. It all takes place in 24 hours. You walk out of the hospital, no wheelchair, no crutches. You realize that you are part of an assembly line. On the day you check-in, Doctor Patel has personally performed your type of operation over 5,000 times. He's clocking them through at a rate of 500 to 700 prostates a year, maybe more. This guy has hit the lottery, and the doctor knows what he's doing. You think he has the best of intentions.

Robotic surgery uses a set of small tools attached to robotic arms. The surgeon controls the robotic arms with the help of a computer. He makes tiny cuts to insert the instruments into your body. An endoscope, a thin tube with a camera at the end of it, lets the surgeon look at enlarged, real-time 3-D images on a large monitor. The robot matches the doctor's hand movements.

Robotic surgeons maintain they can see the procedure better, and work it more precisely, more comfortably. They say they can use the surgical tools much better than with standard endoscopic techniques. They like to tell their detractors that they have taken surgery far beyond the limits of the human hand.

It pisses off Johns Hopkins, the No.1 hospital in America for 21 years in a row. Johns Hopkins Hospital downplays the benefits of robotic surgery, and it does it openly and repeatedly, even suggesting that it may not be a brilliant thing to do. One might expect this from a hospital that prides itself, justifiably, on great surgeons performing excellent, hands-on surgery.

Oddly, Johns Hopkins does have a robotic surgeon on their staff. You never know when a stray prostate will wander over the threshold and demand a little quality time with a robot.

Robotic prostate surgery has become the most common surgery for the treatment of prostate cancer. In February of 2010, The New York Times says it accounts for over 85% of all radical prostatectomies in the United States. The statement might be a reporter's generous stretch of the facts, but not by much.

Florida Hospital Celebration uses the da Vinci robot. They don't hold back on touting the system. Their publicity unabashedly gushes that "the depth of Leonardo da Vinci's unprecedented understanding of human anatomy could likely parallel the sophistication of modern, groundbreaking technology that enables a robotic arm to precisely translate the movements of a surgeon's hands."

That's an embarrassing mouthful as well as a split infinitive. It's enough to alter Leonardo da Vinci's most famous masterpiece, turning Mona Lisa's smile into a frown.

Still, your father taught you to bet on the jockey, not on the horse. Doctor Vipul Patel has personally performed more robotic prostatectomies than anyone else in the world. Make that the Universe. Second place eats his dust, thousands of procedures to the rear (who can resist a quick pun). Now the great doctor is going to take a crack at you (two puns for the price of one).

"I'm in good hands," you tell Kerstin.

"It's a robot," she says.

"Yeah, but the robot is in good hands."

You have only met those hands once, a month or so earlier, in a pre-op meeting with Doctor Patel's assistants. His nurses are all very professional, going through page after page of survey answers that you complete before the operation. The prostate team focuses on avoiding three things: cancer recurrence, incontinence, and impotence.

Suddenly Doctor Patel appears. He is an intense man on a mission, the sort of person who always seems to be in a hurry to reach a distant goal known only to him. Follow the

Leader. The doctor is not the sort of person with whom you have a fireside chat. He is a famous person who will not suffer fools lightly. The doctor is small in stature, but definitely with an above average, take-charge attitude. He stares at you with eyes that burn a bit and tells you everything is going to be okay, and then he disappears. You believe him, and you believe IN him. He is not a person. He is an event.

In the bad old days of prostate removal, doctors chop out your cancerous gland with no regard for the small, fragile, and difficult-to-protect nerves surrounding it.

The nerves handle proper erectile function as well as continence. Radical prostatectomies guarantee life as a eunuch, and a leaking eunuch because diapers are another certainty.

With or without the da Vinci system, doctors today spare many of the nerves they used to dump into bright red bags labeled "Infectious and Pathologic Waste."

Doctor Patel's team seems to consider sexual function as necessary as beating cancer and plugging unintended bladder leaks.

You're talking to a Physician Assistant (PA), Mary Mathe, who reviews all your reports and surveys. Physician Assistants are not full-fledged doctors, but they have usually done six or seven years of science-based post-graduate work. Each state licenses them. The requirements may differ from state to state, but they also need to reregister with their national association every two years, and they need to recertify their license every six years. They do not have to complete residencies for three years (like physicians), but they do train at medical schools and medical centers.

The first employer of PAs is the Veterans Administration (VA) back in 1967. According to the Department of Labor, PA employment is growing much faster than the national average for all occupations.

It will jump almost 30% in the decade starting in 2006. Most of the over 70,000 PAs work in physicians' offices, although 24% work in hospitals. Money Magazine lists PAs as "the fifth-best job in America." PAs in primary care practice make six-digit salaries, and their malpractice insurance costs peanuts (less than $1000) compared to physicians.

Mary Mathe is an attractive blonde with a voice filled with sincere excitement.

She likes what she does for a living (although she will leave the Robotics Institute not long after your operation). She flips pages of medical information.

You've gotten to the sex part.

"After the operation," she says, "you'll sign up for an ED class."

"Who's Ed?" you say. You're going to have some fun with this girl.

"Erectile Dysfunction," she says. You raise your eyebrows, playing stupid with surprise. She's immediately on to you.

"You know all about this," she says with a smile. You think that maybe she's been talking to Kerstin behind your back.

"OK," you say.

"There's a pump you can use after the operation ... not right after, but a few weeks after. You place it over your penis and pump with a handle, and it creates a vacuum that gets your blood flow going, and it helps revive your sexual ability."

You think about this. You put on your best deadpan face. "So, you use this pump to get a hard-on so you can have sex."

She deadpans back. "That's right."

"Will it make Willie grow?"

"Perhaps."

"What happens if you fall in love with the pump?" you ask Mary Mathe, PA.

She deadpans back. "You go blind."

Like doctors and nurses, PAs know too much. They've seen everything, and they've heard all the wisecracks. You laugh. She's good at her job.

Back at Florida Hospital Celebration, you are in the pre-op room where you have received another new catheter before surgery. Kerstin is out in a luxurious waiting room watching television, drinking coffee, reading. Five or six family groups share the space with her, and there's still plenty of room for more.

A patient has gone before you, and you're the second one up to bat. The anesthesiologist gives you some happy juice, and then you are wheeled away, zonked into a dreamless state of darkness. Doctor Patel is in the operating room with his attending physicians, nurses, technicians, and the multi-armed da Vinci robot. There's a lot of plastic covering the machinery, keeping life-threatening bacteria out of the theater of operation.

The da Vinci robot looks like a gigantic mechanical spider with small tools attached to each of its many metal arms.

People wheel you into the middle of the spider. Expert hands make five small incisions across your lower abdomen.

A camera at the end of a thin tube slides into one incision. Everything appears in 3-D on a large, high-definition screen above and to one side of the robot.

For a moment, everything stops.

"I have never seen so much infection," Doctor Patel says the following morning. Your prostate resembles a vast, swollen boil, an enlarged pimple. "This was one of the most difficult surgeries that I have ever performed."

Tiny tools at the end of robotic arms take up their positions through the other incisions in your abdomen.

A drainage tool will keep the operation area clear of blood and other fluids, like a small vacuum cleaner. There are small cutting tools and tiny clamping tools that can stitch and cauterize. They gently push tissues around like little fingers (which they are, since they mimic Doctor Patel's hands, right and left, through the device). The computer even eliminates the slightest hand tremors, breathing life into its "beyond the limits of the human hand" reputation.

One of the attending doctors controls a tiny arm that can offer and withdraw stitching thread. Doctor Patel dissects tissue, isolates the bladder, preserves nerves, cautiously isolates and eliminates the cancerous prostate, and reconnects the bladder.

He puts everything he removes into a small pathological waste bag to withdraw from the body. Another assistant pushes and pulls your catheter on Doctor Patel's command as he stitches your bladder and its connection to the outside world, the urethra, back together.

All of this, of course, is an oversimplification of what the great Doctor does. The skill of the tools matches and magnify the genius of his hands. The tricks he uses just tying a suture seem unbelievable. Doctor Patel has taught hundreds and hundreds of doctors all over the world the near miracle of what he does.

The operation usually takes around two hours. Yours takes almost twice as long.

Kerstin is holding your hand, and you keep telling her that you love her. The fog lifts slowly. You feel no pain.

You immediately know where you are. You suck on some ice. After another 30 minutes, an orderly takes you from the recovery area to your private room. A lot of top resorts in the Caribbean could learn something from this place. It's spacious, friendly, with a great view.

"I hope your room is as good as this one," you tell Kerstin. She's staying at a local hotel within walking distance of the hospital. She tries to get into the Bohemian, a famous place attached to the Florida Hospital, but no room is available. Florida Hospital is a bustling place.

"Want to go down to the pool and have a drink?" you ask. "This is just a one-night stand, you know." You feel pretty good.

"The only thing you're going to get up for is your first walk in a few hours," she says. She can be adamant, this Viking woman, but you can tell by the smile in her eyes that she's happy to see you alive. You doze off.

A nurse wakes you, and it's time to walk around the track, a circuit of several hundred yards that passes all the patient rooms on the floor. Kerstin is on one side of you and the nurse on the other.

You make it. "Another," you say as you approach the door to your room, showing off — tough guy. The second circuit almost brings you to your knees. You get back into bed slowly, and the nurse says you can make the circuit any time, but ring for assistance first. If they don't see you on the floor, they will come and drag you out of bed. She reminds you a little of your Marine Corps Drill Instructor back in the early 60s, although he did not have a mustache (I am just kidding, of course).

Kerstin leaves for the hotel. She'll be back in the morning. Three times during the night, you make the circuit, twice around every time. Then you doze off immediately after completing each marathon.

Suddenly, half a dozen doctors surround you, all looking at you with serious expressions on their faces. For a second, you think you're dreaming, or you've gone to the Hospital in Hell.

Doctor Patel is at the foot of your bed, slightly in front of all the other physicians. It's real. He tells you about the enormous infection you had and how this was perhaps his most difficult robotic prostatectomy.

"How do you feel?" he asks.

"You want to arm wrestle?" you answer. Your voice cracks a little, groggy as you speak. He smiles, but not with his eyes. None of the doctors around him reacts. You all stare at each other for a moment.

"You are a great doctor," you say. "Thank you for being a great doctor, and thank you for being my doctor." Suddenly everyone is nodding, and the room finally relaxes.

"All of the infection is gone now," Doctor Patel promises you.

"I got all of it."

He nods and then the entire entourage washes out the door in a wave of starched white jackets and gleaming new stethoscopes.

Kerstin arrives and watches you eat a simple breakfast.

You discuss the death of your infection and the remarkable brilliance of Doctor Patel. You run a few more marathons around the circuit, moving your pace up from a wobbling garden snail to a geriatric turtle. You feel good. You check out of the resort. You stop at the pharmacy on the ground floor to pick up some prescriptions and absorbent diapers. You head back to Boca.

You will return in a week for a post-op session with the team and then again a few weeks later for some follow-up courses on incontinence and sex. You have already received a lot of information for those classes.

The first post-op will include the dreaded removal of your catheter, which scares both of you. Will the plumbing work?

They will also check your PSA rating to see if the cancer is gone.

The week passes slowly. You walk a lot and gradually raise your stamina to a little over a mile, the distance from your house to the community's security gate, and back again. You often glance at the small pool separating the two buildings in your courtyard home, which has a main house and a guest house. You have not been in the pool for over three months because of your constant catheterization. The risk of infection keeps you high and dry. In retrospect, it does not seem to make much difference. You still reach the top of Doctor Patel's "infected prostate" list.

You drive back up to Celebration and check into the hotel Kerstin stayed at during your surgery. You walk over to the hospital and enter a different building, where Doctor Patel has his urology office. It looks like Doctor Gottenger's office, a little more crowded, but the same waiting lounge.

The people who work in Doctor Patel's office, however, treat patients like friends instead of "next in line." There's free bottled water, packages of nuts, and pretzels.

You know that if you have to use the bathroom, you won't have to threaten to break through the door.

Many doctors do not understand marketing. They are slaves to their craft. They perform whatever field of medicine they specialize in, and they expect a thankful world to beat a path to their door. Since their offices lead to continued health, they often get away with second-rate staff and structures.

Smart patients, Warrior Patients, judge doctors based on their weakest links: receptionists who don't care, technicians who watch the clock instead of patients, nurses who are sick of sick people, and office systems that confuse everyone.

Any or all of these can scalpel the best intentions of a doctor. Doctor Patel understands this as well as he understands the precise art of robotic surgery.

You and Kerstin enter an examination room. After a quick battery of questions, the nurse takes your catheter tube and pumps sterilized water into it.

You begin to feel uncomfortable, queasy as your bladder fills up. Then the nurse slowly pulls the plug. Your bladder empties without the catheter, which is something it has not done for many months.

"That's great," she says. "A lot more came out than went in."

"What does that mean?" you ask.

Kerstin is already smiling. The nurse gives you an answer, and you laugh.

With your pants still down around your ankles, you slide off the examination chair and hug her. Then you hug Kerstin. You repeat what the nurse has told you.

"The plumbing is working just fine."

Doctor Patel appears shortly after this. He glances at the information on a clipboard. He says: "Your PSA is less than zero point one." The readout shows ">0.1," and the Doctor tells you it does not go lower than that.

They will monitor you over the coming years, but the cancer is gone.

"I am cancer-free," you say.

He nods. Everyone smiles. The town of Celebration has lived up to its name. Doctor Patel has lived up to his.

You do mention to him that you still feel a little infected. His eyes lock onto yours.

"The infection is no longer there," he says. His eyes seem fierce. "It is gone."

Let it be so.

You drive around Celebration looking for swimming trunks, find a bright green pair that brings out the Irish in you and return to your hotel. You go swimming, a joy you have not felt for many months. Blue Florida skies, laughter, hugging in the pool, warm water washing over your cancer-free body. It is as good as it gets.

In two weeks, you will return to join some of your fellow graduates from the Global Robotics Institute of Florida Hospital. It will be an eye-opening gathering for both Kerstin and yourself.

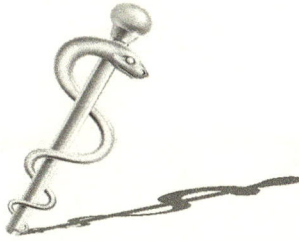

<u>Warrior Patient Rule 4</u>: People usually think their doctor is the best in the world, even if their doctor is in the process of burying them. Trust but verify, also outstanding doctors. Your life will depend on it.

Chapter 5

A Growing Business

im**potence**

They are looking at Mary as the scoffer spits: "It don't work worth a damned!"

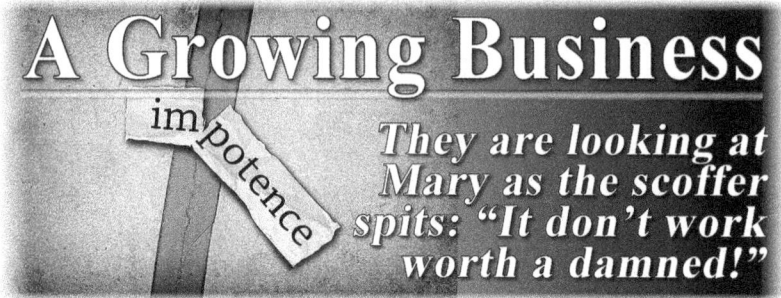

As a business, erectile dysfunction (ED) is not limping along. Unlike its victims, it's growing. You and Kerstin sit in a classroom at the Florida Hospital, and she is enthralled by what she is learning about the male species.

Mary Mathe, PA, leads the ED Class. Family and friends applaud her as the person who suggests you might go blind if you fall in love with a suction pump.

The name of the class has a catchy title, "Erectile Dysfunction and Penile Rehabilitation." Privately, you interpret this as meaning that if it stays limp, it goes to jail, but perhaps you don't have that quite right.

A week after your robotic radical prostatectomy, you send an e-mail to your sons, brothers, sister, her husband, Ed Baumheier (who always has useful advice and stories to relate), nieces, nephews, friends, and the President of the United States announcing that you are "cancer-free" and qualified to wear a blue ribbon "survivor" pin on your lapel. Your e-mail says:

It looks like I am cancer-free, and will recover to most normal levels of activity in about 4-5 weeks.

If you don't want all the details, with a small sprinkling of humor, you can stop here and just accept my thanks for your love and support throughout this process.

Most of the men should probably read on, however, because like it or not, if you get old enough, you will probably enjoy and hopefully survive a similar experience.

Here's what the Doctor wrote in the surgical pathology report.

My Gleason score going into the operation was 3+4=7. They thought it might be 4+3=7, which sums the same, but which would have meant a far higher likelihood that the carcinoma (cancer) had spread more now than the prostate.

Five percent of my prostate had a cancerous tumor. The organ was about twice the size of one's healthy prostate, and it was entirely covered by "exuberant necrotizing granulomatous" inflammation. (My translation: the original prostate biopsy was performed by Genghis Khan with a steam shovel and got infected as hell.)

The diagnosis during and after surgery showed that the surgical resection margins were tumor-free. So were the lymph nodes. The bladder neck was tumor-free, the bilateral pelvic nodes were benign and tumor-free, and the resection margins were tumor-free. The extraprostatic extension was absent, and seminal vesicle invasion was also gone.

That's a bunch of fancy writing that suggests the operation was a 100% success. I was on my feet and walked a mile 36 hours after the surgery. The catheter is finally gone, and the river flows downstream (for the first time in 4 months).

Last night I slept on my stomach for the first time in 4 months.

Yesterday I swam in our pool for the first time in 4 months.

I am learning Kegel exercises, which should return me to a state of continence within a month or two. Women understand Kegel exercises, but many men don't; it strengthens the pelvic floor muscles to the point where a good sneeze, a cough, or just leaning over does not cause leakage.

It might take me a couple of months' worth of diapers to regain my control.

There are about 60 million men in America with erectile dysfunction, and any prostatectomy guarantees you join their ranks. For a start.

But the robotic approach I chose through the gifted hands of Doctor Patel gives me a fighting chance to escape.

My operation only destroyed about 10% of the cavernous nerves responsible for proper function. That's normal when you cut out the prostate. Ten years ago, they just sliced and diced, and 100% of the nerves suffered the scalpel. You had no chance of a healthy sex life after that. No one knew. Now they do.

For four weeks, Kerstin and I have to abstain from all attempts at sex. It can take up to a year, but I have about a 90% chance of successfully attacking the woman I love regularly.

There is even a device that helps me along the way (I can't use it for four more weeks). It's a hand-operated vacuum pump that you have to use daily until your gear shift usually operates.

My doctor told me it worked well.

Kerstin and I have decided that the device needs a name. We chose one of our favorite Russian tennis stars: Suckalot Oritsova (that's a joke; no such lady on the courts).

Anyway, the OPERATION WAS A SUCCESS, THE PATIENT LIVED, I AM CANCER-FREE, AND I WILL WORK HARD TO BECOME NORMAL AGAIN (well, normal is relative, I guess, but you know what I mean).

Thanks to all of you for your good wishes and prayers. We could not have done it without you.

The White House never responds. Everyone else does, including your sister's husband, Ed, who once had a catheter for an enlarged prostate. He previously sympathized with your problems in that area by suggesting that you consult the oil and gas tycoon, T. Boone Pickens. Most people know that Mr. Pickens has established himself as a world-class expert on pipelines. God bless friends and laughter; two of the most powerful medicines in the world.

Now you and Kerstin return to Florida Hospital in Celebration for post-op education. Mary Mathe, PA, uses a PowerPoint presentation on a large screen at the front of the class. About

30 people attend, many of them spouses and girlfriends. You meet some of them out in the hallway before class, and they seem very angry, which surprises both you and Kerstin. You are happy with the surgery and the results. At least so far.

"Erectile dysfunction is the persistent inability to have or keep an erection firm enough for sex," Mary tells us, and she has the PowerPoint slide to prove it. She has made this presentation often, and she moves smoothly in front of the class, smiling, making her point, and never touching her perfect blonde hair. It does not flutter at all as Mary moves back and forth in her starched white doctor's jacket. She is a pro, and she knows her onions.

"An estimated 20 to 30 million men in America have erectile dysfunction with varying degrees of severity," she tells the class. "You are not alone." In your mind, you visualize a massive army of men, limping along.

Years earlier, you made a living in the presentation business. Mary Mathe, PA, has excellent slides, with information sources in small type along the bottom and the Florida Hospital logo in the lower right-hand corner of each one. A tasteful blue border matches the color of the logo perfectly.

Mary talks about two types of erectile dysfunction. The psychogenic and the medically challenged. The psychogenic men suffer from depression or relationship issues, and age, while the medical contingent faces the problems of prostate cancer treatment or high blood pressure or diabetes. There are no clear lines and men can put their, uh, feet in both groups.

The classroom starts to fidget a little, smelling too much psycho-babble.

Mary shows everyone the anatomy of an erection. The classroom calms down, but Kerstin seems spellbound by the cavernous nerves traveling down the lower spine and surrounding the prostate gland.

A squeak of a laugh escapes from you as you watch her (God you love this woman), and some people turn and glare in your direction. You mouth "sorry" and immediately turn your attention back to Mary and the screen.

Mary's slide shows an almost surreal, limp penis, something Salvatore Dali might melt onto a canvas along with a clock. On the screen, the illustration strips away the outer tissues, and Mary talks about good arterial blood flow and good venous blood flow for an erection to occur. In ED cases, blood flow is restricted, often by vascular diseases. That causes between 50% and 70% of ED problems. Kerstin is taking a lot of notes.

The presentation discusses the natural chemicals in the body that lead to erections. Then Mary shows a slide of Prostate Cancer Treatment Options: Surgery, radiation, cryotherapy, HIFU (an acronym for High Intensity Focused Ultrasound, which uses sound energy to zap cancerous tissue in the prostate without harming nearby tissue), hormonal treatment, and watchful waiting (doing nothing).

All of which seems a bit moot to you since every man in the room has taken a ride on Doctor Patel's assembly line and had a robotic radical prostatectomy.

Perhaps a few of the people still sit on the fence considering the procedure.

However, you do not meet any of them before the class starts.

Maybe some of the people are unlucky, and they need additional treatment for cancer spreading to other parts of their bodies.

"There are major risk factors you can modify or change with lifestyle adjustments or medication," Mary tells us. Stop smoking. Don't do street drugs. Control cholesterol and blood pressure. Exercise. Lose the tube around the middle of your body. It's all pretty obvious stuff. There's one scruffy dude in the class who looks like he might be doing street drugs, but you never know.

Then Mary gives a plug for the "nerve-sparing" technique of robot-assisted radical prostatectomies. Must be some holdouts in the room. Then she slips in a warning that even with better surgery, a man's natural sex function is unlikely to heal if left alone.

You could hear a pin drop. Seats creak. The warning is not what the patients want to believe before the robot peels their grape. The skilled hands of Doctor Patel promise a quick return to connubial and, if so inclined, non-connubial bliss. A lot of people in the class didn't read the fine print, yourself included.

"Why does it take so long?" Mary asks. A PowerPoint slide slips onto the screen with three answers: post-operative inflammation, mechanical nerve stretching, and reduced oxygenation leading to scarring. At the bottom of the slide, two small black ant-like creatures pull a green ribbon between them. It might be a nerve. It might be a tape measure.

Nobody asks.

You skip to treatment options, which are Sildenafil (Viagra®), Vardenafil (Levitra®), and Tadalafil (Cialis®). Non-drugs include intra-urethral suppositories and penile injections. You can start oral medication after they remove your catheter as long as you're not taking nitroglycerin.

Kerstin has been scribbling studiously on a handout of the presentation.

A PowerPoint slide flashes: "Take it before you go to bed."

You consider this a great double entendre. You point it out to Kerstin with a chuckle. More people glare in your direction.

You think you might be sitting in the middle of an uptight group of dissatisfied psychogenic customers.

Finally, Mary gets to the penis vacuum device, which I have privately named Suckalot Oritsova, my favorite imaginary Russian tennis player. Kerstin protests at the moniker, but she cannot subdue my tasteless sense of humor. You can start having a meaningful relationship with the pump four weeks after surgery. Every day for 10 minutes, for up to a year. The slide ends with an all-caps warning and three exclamation points: "NO INTERCOURSE BEFORE 4 WEEKS POST OP!!!"

The man behind you scoffs loudly. He has been fidgeting in his chair, waiting to pounce, and you are delighted to relinquish your crown as the "glare at" person.

Only nobody is glaring at him. They are looking at Mary as the scoffer spits: "It don't work worth a damned!" You were never sure about the pronunciation of "worth a damned," but it apparently ends with a hard "d" because the man emphasizes it clearly and with a lot of power.

And Mary Mathe, PA, handles it adeptly, asking him to explain the problem.

He's a good-looking man, more dignified than his manners, but he's outraged. His significant other sits next to him.

She has sharp eyes and a supportive sneer on her pinched face. She'd look a lot better if she didn't do that. She might even inspire her partner to try harder.

The man says: "I've been using the pump for a month, and it does not work. It does not form a proper vacuum."

Now, admittedly you don't know anything about these pumps. You have not seen one yet in real life, although there's a small illustration of a plastic tube device on the screen. You think maybe this guy has stumbled into a sticky trap.

Mary's going to tell him to get a smaller, tighter tube. Instead, Mary asks how he uses it. You have the feeling she has been here before.

It turns out he has been using a sex-enhancement ointment with the vacuum pump. You keep a straight face, but visions of this guy walking down the aisle in a marriage ceremony to Suckalot Oritsova makes the edges of your mouth twitch a little. Mary points out that he can't use that sort of ointment with the penis pump. He needs to use a lotion with higher viscosity. The fluid he has been using excites women. She leaves it at that and does not add "vacuum pumps don't care."

Now his partner's sneer, sharp eyes, and pinched face are directed at the dummy with whom she's living. He shrugs awkwardly and says, "Thank you." The moment passes.

The PowerPoint presentation is winding down. A photo of two cute little dogs on a couch under the title PENILE REHABILITATION pops up and suggests, "If there is a partner, INVOLVE THEM! Their involvement is CRITICAL in your recovery!"

You have a hard time wrapping your mind around rehabilitation without a partner's involvement unless you want to go blind, but you get what they mean. You do need to talk about it.

A final slide slips onto the screen with the heading: "QUESTIONS???" Below that is a photo close-up of a plant that looks almost exactly like a giant, swollen penis. It's growing out of the stony desert soil, some variety of cactus. The room stares at it, silent. Then everyone bursts into laughter. Uproarious, relieving laughter. You can do it. You can make it. And Mary knows her stuff.

Very few people ask questions, and most of them want to know where they can get the pump. Not so amazingly, there is a pump salesman right there at the show, hiding in the back of the classroom.

He steps forward and does a brisk business. Once again, you remind yourself that you are part of the Global Robotics Institute's assembly line. Doctor Patel has hit the lottery, and he knows what he's doing.

Next up: "Urinary Incontinence" with a much-needed break for all the incontinent ticket-holders. The men crush each other into the hallway and race for the toilets. You are surprised and relieved that Doctor Patel's bean counters have not yet invaded the facilities; they are not toilets demanding an entry fee.

Another Physician Assistant, a dark-haired, serious woman named Christan Martone, PA, handles the Urinary Incontinence show. Like Mary Mathe, PA, she also no longer works at the Robotics Institute in Celebration, Florida.

Christan's presentation starts with a dog sniffing a fluffy white toy. You have no idea why. Perhaps it is a secret method of housebreaking puppies and leaking grown-ups.

The next PowerPoint slide says that we are not alone and points out that we suffer from the most common side effect of a prostatectomy. The slide contains an illustration of a leaking faucet. It also has good news: "98% of men will regain their urinary control!!!!!" I'm not sure it needs five exclamation points, but, indeed, you can never emphasize good news enough.

The next slide has a three-dimensional chart that shows five blue columns growing from just under 70% after six weeks up to 98% after a year and a half. You decide to place yourself in the first column. After three weeks, your leaky faucet appears almost normal.

You have been doing Kegel exercises religiously. You are probably coming to that part of the show, you think.

There are two kinds of incontinence: stress and urge. Kerstin leans over to you and whispers that women understand the stress type better than men. "That's because men don't pay attention to stress," you whisper back. "We're tougher." She smiles at you patiently.

Stress incontinence means you have leakage because of laughing, sneezing, coughing, or other physical stressors on the abdominal cavity and, therefore, the bladder.

You whisper to your wife, Kerstin, that you had no idea that they were talking about that sort of stress.

She smiles at you patiently.

Urge incontinence, Christan Martone explains, is the "I gotta go, I gotta go" syndrome.

"That's what I have," you tell Kerstin, your whisper a bit louder.

You do not look at her, but you know that she is smiling at you, patiently.

Stress incontinence is a pelvic floor issue. Men do not understand the pelvic floor. They have a fire hose that they can turn on and off with a squeeze, a jiggle, and a shake.

Once we are housebroken as children, we learn to step up to the urinals of life with high confidence and ability. Some of us may have bashful bladders in a busy toilet area such as ballparks, but the fire hose can usually operate on automatic.

Women are different, marvelously different. They recognize, at an early age, the dangers of sneezing, laughing, and coughing. They use Kegel exercises to cut down on life's little mistakes.

Every man who has a prostatectomy realizes, immediately, that laughter is no longer a laughing matter.

Sneezes produce results well beyond the nasal passages. Coughs usually end with an apologetic "whoops."

Christan Martone, PA, launches into Kegel exercises. She remains very serious, talking to a room filled with puppies in need of housebreaking.

You hope she does not give Kerstin permission to swat you with the newspaper when you make a mistake.

That's what your father and mother do with the Labrador puppies the family breeds when you are a teenager, and it works without fail on every litter our blonde Lab, Olive has. Your father gives Olive that name because she descends from a well-documented thoroughbred named "Gin" via a bitch named "Martini."

Doctor Arnold Kegel develops his namesake exercises in the 1940s in Los Angeles, where he is a gynecologist.

Kegel exercises strengthen vaginal muscles after childbirth.

In women, the exercises shorten, tighten and rehabilitate the muscles stretching from the front of the pelvis around the rectum. Later, when radical prostatectomies become common for men with prostate cancer, doctors discover that Kegel exercises also strengthen the muscles that control a man's urinary stream. Doctor Kegel becomes the champion of self-restraint among men.

Christan works through two new PowerPoint slides, both with three bullet points on them. But the bullet points are not small circles; they are little drips. Cute touch. Florida Hospital is full of pros.

Kegel exercises strengthen the pelvic floor muscles. You find them when you stop and start your urine stream.

It's mental. You need to feel your lower abdomen tighten up, on the inside, not on your abs. Once you isolate the right muscle with a small cerebral "eureka moment," you can start working the muscle. The easiest way is to squeeze and hold your urine stream for five to ten seconds. Release. Hold. Release. Hold. Ten times. That's one set. You'll run out of urine before you run out of repetitions.

It is not easy. You need to do thirty sets, three hundred repetitions, every single day. If you get sore, and you will, then decrease the hold time. But do the reps, at least if you want to join the dry brigade.

Urge incontinence usually relates to the size of your prostate and often requires medicine and further medical procedures. But if you've had a radical prostatectomy, urge incontinence probably will not occur.

Christan Martone starts to wind up the urinary incontinence show with a PowerPoint slide of "Tips and Tricks."

Avoid bladder irritants like coffee, citrus juice, and alcohol. You turn into a teetotaler half a year before your prostate biopsy, not because you have to, but because you know nobody in your family who benefits from booze after they reach their late sixties. And you see a bunch of them whose lives are wrecked by it. You also notice your balance is not as right as it used to be, especially with a drink in your hand.

Balance improves after you ditch the alcohol. Plus, you always know where your car is parked when you wake up in the morning.

You do miss Guinness, which you consider to be the fifth food group in any adequately balanced diet.

You stop drinking cold turkey, the same way Kerstin and you give up smoking 35 years earlier. She still enjoys a glass of wine every day, but you are alcohol-free. You enjoy parties and laughter and fun, and you make no judgment on others who like to juice things up with a drink.

The Tips and Tricks slide's next secret is "Wear darker pants," which gets a laugh from a few of the guys.

And avoid wearing boxers, because there are no commandos in the High and Dry Brigade.

The show ends with a slide of a small figurine peeing into a fountain. A lot of men laugh, and a lot of men don't.

The women like it.

A tough-looking guy in the front row, who has been chatting up Kerstin out in the hall between shows, holds up a pair of newly acquired diapers.

They have frills on them. Catcalls and whistles end the gathering with laughter.

As you are getting up to leave, you look at a leather-faced guy behind you and say: "Sounds like a piece of cake."

"Bullcrap," he answers.

He is not a joyful person. He looks old and drained.

You think maybe he is a Panhandle farmer who has lost his tan, spending too much time in doctors' waiting rooms. If you follow all the instructions, you tell him you think you can make it all right.

"How long since your operation?" he asks you.

"Three weeks."

"You don't know jack-shit!" he tells you.

He turns and slumps out of the room, with a small, silent woman in his wake. You and Kerstin are both taken by surprise.

You have no idea how close to the truth this fellow has gotten.

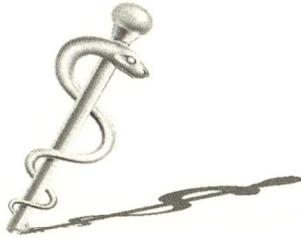

<u>Warrior Patient Rule 5</u>: Cut down on bad habits. Don't smoke, even if you're on fire. Ditch drinking (one glass of wine a day, but no more). Your balance gets much better, in every respect.

Chapter 6

"Come Home."

You feel numb. You put your feet on the floor and freeze. Your lower body is covered with blood blisters.

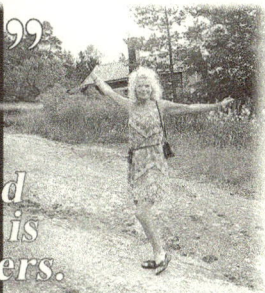

After six weeks, you have beaten incontinence.

You can sneeze and cough without springing a leak.

You play tennis, always early in the morning and never more than one set.

You try a little golf, making sure you limit it to nine holes late in the day.

You also get severe night sweats for the first time in your life. Your side of the bed is soaked every morning.

In men, night sweats can mean many things, from nothing to simple Andropause (male menopause), to a list of unpleasant, often deadly diseases.

Cialis can cause night sweats, which you take to get Willie to stand at attention.

So far, he remains at parade rest.

Every time you step into the shower, the penis pump joins you. It's a lot less fun than you thought it would be, in fact, a bit painful.

Willie always responds, but not long enough to make it from the bathroom to the bedroom. He seems to die whenever he gets ten feet from the shower.

There's an elastic band that can put a stranglehold on Willie. It keeps blood in the penis, but Kerstin widens her eyes and giggles at Willie singing the blues, a very bright blue, which makes you laugh as well. And the elastic band is killing you. It doesn't work.

You keep taking Cialis; you keep showering with the penis pump, and you keep having night sweats. Your new front-loading washer and dryer work overtime on bed linens

One morning, in the shower after tennis, you push the pump a little more than usual. Willie's resistance to change frustrates you. Something snaps in your groin.

You hit the release button, making the vacuum vanish, but the pain takes almost an hour to go away.

It does disappear, however, although there is a sheet of hardness in your lower left abdomen that you never felt before.

Within two months, a hernia will start popping out.

Another common cause of night sweats is an infection, perhaps the most common cause, and you think that some sort of disease remains in your body. You can feel it. You know it's there. You keep waiting for your immune system to take care of it.

One of your best friends, Brian Greenman, tells his wife, Judy: "You know, Temple is starting to walk like an old man."

A shuffle invades the typical spring in your steps, but you tell yourself you are getting old. You're a little out of shape. You spend too much time on your butt in front of computer screens.

You're a Real Estate Broker, with a corporate Brokerage (Templeworks Properties, LLC), and you have not sold a house, or even shown one, for a long time. You want to get back to the business after six months of illness. You own several dozen websites. You need to get them working again. They help home buyers and sellers make smart decisions, and you enjoy real estate. You're good at it. Your health has stopped you from doing it and continues to do so. It's also a rotten housing market, close to the bottom after the great Housing Bubble, which burst four years earlier.

There's a dull, constant weight in your lower back. Brian Greenman gives you a book on back pain. You read it cover to cover and do many of the exercises it recommends. The dull, lethargic, slightly queasy discomfort remains.

Your eyesight seems to be deteriorating as well, and the world takes on a dull hue. It affects your left eye the most. You can't see a tennis ball clearly, and sometimes you close your left eye and try to concentrate on the yellow ball with just your good one. One of your best childhood friends, Brian Jerome, had his eye poked out by his sister, a tragic accident. Blind in one eye, he still plays great tennis. You can never beat him.

One morning you look at your tennis partners and say: "I thought we were going to use new balls."

"They are new," they say.

"They look old." You roll one in your hand, bounce it on the court with your racket.

"I just opened the can," Lee Gelfond tells you. That proves it because Lee always likes to play with brand new balls. But these balls have lost their bright yellow color. All of them look used, although they bounce new.

Nobody else seems to have a problem with them.

Your better eye starts to get a bit foggier. Not bad. Just a little.

You'll be fine.

Driving at night becomes difficult.

Kerstin has a summer trip planned to Scandinavia. The Swedish women are gathering again to celebrate their roots, their language, their traditions, their womanhood. It's called the Swedish Women's Educational Association (SWEA). You refer to it, with humor, as the Swedish Mafia, but the women grow tired of this, so you don't say it too often. Omerta (silence).

Kerstin joins SWEA women once or twice a year in different parts of the world. Morocco. China. Turkey. Greece. Sicily. Italy. Spain. Israel.

And each year, many SWEA return to Sweden, discovering different parts of their homeland during the time of the midnight sun.

You tell your friends that you don't mind Kerstin leaving for two- and three-week trips a few times a year. "As long as she comes back home. Alone."

"You cannot trap a butterfly and expect it to keep its bright colors," you say. You say it often, and you mean it.

This year Kerstin is going to Västergötland (West Gothland) to "Walk in the Footsteps of Arn Magnusson," a Knight Templar born in that area in 1150. Arn Magnusson is a fictional character, the creation of Swedish author Jan Guillou. The SWEA women follow the footsteps of the fictional hero in Guillou's famous Crusades Trilogy. The Knight Templar is a thread that guides a busload of 50 SWEA women through the southwestern landskap (province) of Västergötland. They travel through wooded uplands and lakes, past rocky ridges that rise to elevations of 1,000 feet, to a church over 1000 years old, and a castle originally built-in 1298. Only a small portion of the province's area touches the sea, but it includes Gothenburg, Sweden's second-largest city, and an important port. Kerstin is born in Gothenburg.

SWEA started in Los Angeles in 1979. It now has almost 8,000 members in over 70 chapters in 33 different countries.

Kerstin was the President of the New York Chapter when you lived in SOHO in Manhattan, and briefly the President of the South Florida Chapter when you moved to Boca Raton.

It's a wonderful non-profit organization, and they do good things with scholarships and cultural events.

Whenever dozens of SWEA women get together, they always increase the weight and volume of laughter in the world.

"Are you going to be all right?" Kerstin asks you.

"I'll be fine," you say. "Go. Have a great time. Say 'hi' to Sweden for me. And remember to come back."

You live in Sweden for two winters, a few years after you marry, long enough to speak the language poorly. Sweden is a beautiful country filled with beautiful people. The darkness of winter eventually drives you back to America.

Kerstin smiles, but she is worried about leaving you. So are you. Whenever you are apart, you always text each other. If something goes wrong, you will send a secret message that says, "Come Home."

You drive her to Miami Airport. You feel a hint of deep sadness as you return home alone, but she will never know.

Whatever problem you have will go away. You are cancer-free. You will be good as new when the love of your life returns in three weeks. You will make love and laugh and shout like teenagers in the grip of raging hormones.

You'll get all of Templeworks' websites going and list a bunch of homes and sell them, and everything will be fine. You book an appointment with the eye doctor. You have not had your eyes examined for almost ten years.

You also need to make an appointment to see your primary doctor at Personal Physician Care. You need to deal with your constant back pain. You have mixed feelings about Doctor Susan Barish.

Not because she fires the starting gun with a snap of the rubber glove at your annual physical six months earlier.

No, it is because she refers you to Doctor Gottenger.

In your household, the doctor has a name, fairly or unfairly, of Genghis Khan with a steam shovel. After all, it was his prostate biopsy that brought out the infection in you, and he does nothing beyond saying to you: "I wonder why you're so infected."

You consider making an appointment at the Florida Hospital in Celebration. You trust Doctor Patel and his team. Maybe they should take a look at you. But you have a hard time driving a car for four hours with all the pain in your lower back.

Your doubts about Doctor Susan Barish remain. You think back to Kerstin's false alarm with ovarian cancer.

It was a referral from Doctor Barish, which sent her to the doctor's office that gave her, and you such a scare.

And another referral from Doctor Barish, for a second opinion, sent her to a doctor who tried to sign her up for immediate surgery.

At a dinner at a close friend's house, you meet a doctor who has worked at Personal Physician Care.

The dinner is at Daphne Loewendahl's home, across the street in our subdivision.

Daphne makes her living as a concert pianist, working under the stage name of Daphne Spottiswoode.

She wins a scholarship to the Royal Academy of Music in London.

She studies in Paris.

Daphne becomes a prize-winner at an international competition in Geneva.

She is famous on the BBC and a soloist on many cruise lines over the years.

She is a guest soloist with all the major British orchestras and often featured on British and American television.

She's a delightful neighbor and close friend who regularly treats Kerstin and yourself to the world's best Sheppard's Pie.

One night you walk into Daphne's home and shake hands with a pleasant, good-looking blonde lady, a doctor.

You start talking about health, and that leads to the story of Kerstin's troubling referrals.

"Oh," the doctor says, "I used to work at Personal Physician Care."

"You don't work there now?" you ask.

"Didn't like the way they did things," she says. "Every night before I left my office, I would make sure I had read all my e-mails from patients. I responded to every one of them before leaving."

She shrugs.

More is coming. "I think I was the only doctor there who did it. They had hundreds of questions from patients that they just disregarded. Or messages that they never answered. A lot of messages never even got through the assistants to the doctors."

She speaks about surprising patient disregard and a severe lack of attention to detail. "They have dozens of e-mails from patients every day that they never answer," she repeats. She leaves the clinic and works elsewhere.

Kerstin decides that Personal Physician Care, where Doctor Susan Barish shares offices with six other doctors, will no longer be her Primary Physician. She switches to the Cleveland Clinic.

But you like Doctor Barish. And the convenience of a five-minute drive to Personal Physician Care outweighs a long and very tiresome four-hour journey to the Florida Hospital in Celebration.

You make an appointment to see Doctor Barish the next day.

Personal Physician Care leases satellite office space near The Delray Community Hospital. Every medical center in America spawns such offices. They all look relatively similar: waiting room, reception area, fake and real plants, a television on the wall which most people ignore, a door that regularly opens as a nurse or assistant calls out the name of a waiting patient. Disappear through the door, step on a weight scale, get your blood pressure taken, and wait for the doctor.

At the reception desk, they tell you that Doctor Barish is not available, although the appointment you make is with her.

"Doctor Barish is in Europe with her family," a girl behind a sliding glass barrier says. She does not look at you, but rather at a notepad in front of her. "Your appointment is with Doctor Abreu."

You have no idea who that is, but you work on the pronunciation of his name: Ah-BREY-You.

"I hope nothing is wrong," you say.

She looks up.

"Oh no, he's an excellent doctor."

"I mean with Doctor Barish. I hope everyone in the family is OK." She stares at you. Such knowledge is apparently above her pay grade. She tells you what the co-pay is, and you hand her your credit card. They don't take that credit card any longer, so you give her another one. Then you sit in an uncomfortable seat and wait to be called.

Doctor Manuel Abreu is in his mid-forties, attractive, soft-spoken, with a stethoscope around his neck and a nicely starched white doctor's jacket. He reads some information about you on the computer screen in the examination room and tells you that you're neighbors. He also lives at the Boca Country Club, in a subdivision called The Greens. You and Kerstin live in Mykonos Court, just one community and less than half a mile away. He has kids and has recently moved in. You are bonding, but something tells you that you're going to stick with Doctor Susan Barish when she returns.

Doctor Abreu thinks a seven-day dose of Cipro will fix you. He agrees that you have some sort of infection.

You tell him you think you should have a workup, and he orders a blood test. "We'll do it in a few weeks," he says. You ask when Doctor

Barish will return, and he does not know. He gets a urine sample from you. He writes a prescription, and you shake hands, pleasant neighbors, saying "adios."

You stop taking the Cialis, but the night sweats continue. When you bathe, the pump remains on the shower floor. The hardness in your groin prevents you from freeing Willie in a vacuum. With Kerstin overseas in Sweden, what's the point?

A week later, you are back with Doctor Abreu. Your pain has gotten worse. Your body starts to crumple up. He consults his computer and searches for another answer to your agony. He settles on a drug called Diclofenac, 75 mg for the pain. He calls in the prescription to the pharmacy at Costco, across the road from the Boca Country Club, where you all live. You can pick it up in an hour or two. Doctor Abreu does not attempt to examine you, and you never remove your shirt. His stethoscope remains neatly tucked around his neck. You simply sit there and get a prescription.

He's a pill pusher.

When you get to the pharmacy at 4 o'clock, the prescription is not ready. It has not registered on their computer. They double-check. They call Personal Physician Care, and everything gets sorted out after about thirty minutes.

They hand you the prescription.

You are in pain, and you go home hoping for a miracle drug. You do not even look at what they have given you.

You open the package. It's a five-day supply of Cipro, not Diclofenac.

You return to Costco, but the pharmacy is closed. You struggle back home. You need to make it to the next day to get the right stuff.

You return to Costco the next morning, first in line, when they slide up the rolling shutters on the main entrance at 10 o'clock. You hope that the correct prescription, for Diclofenac, has arrived. It has not.

It is Thursday, and the pharmacist phones Personal Physician Care, trying his best to sort out the problem.

He cannot get through to Doctor Abreu. He says he will send an e-mail to them, and maybe it will be ready later in the day. You start to take the Cipro.

The pharmacy is about to close when you return for the Diclofenac. Nothing has come from Personal Physicians Care. You go home. You consider stopping by Doctor Abreu's home in the Greens. As a licensed Real Estate Broker, you can find out where Doctor Abreu lives in thirty seconds on one of your computers. You decide not to invade Doctor Abreu's privacy. He does not seem all that interested in helping you.

You send Kerstin a text message about the prescription fiasco. You try to turn the prescription foul-up into a comedy of errors. You tell her you're OK. You love her.

She sees right through this and texts: "Do you want me to come home?"

"No," you text back. "Have fun. I'm OK. I'm fine."

You curl up in bed, watch television, and sweat a lot. You have two cats, and they are both on the bed. Truffles curls up at your feet. HiJinks rolls on his back, fluffy and soft, paws up, and feet splayed. You want to be a cat in Kerstin's house in your next life. You hope it does not come too soon. You sleep.

When you wake up, you dial the number for Personal Physicians Care, and, after a lot of time, you leave a message for the Doctor on Call. You say they have screwed up your pain prescription, and you hurt a lot. He calls back and asks you what the medicine is.

"It's for pain," you say.

"No," he says. "What is the medication?"

You have to look at a piece of paper on which you have written "Diclofenac."

"Diclofenac Sodium," he says, but differently — dye-KLOE-fen-ack SOE-dee-um — correcting your layman's pronunciation.

He pauses, then adds: "I'm sorry, but I don't know you ."

"Well," you answer, "I'm a nice guy, six foot one and a half, about 215 pounds, ex-Marine, ex-New York City Cop, ex-Reader's Digest Editor, ex-...." He suddenly interrupts your fourth "ex-."

"Yah-yah," he says dismissively. "What I mean is that I can't prescribe any pain medication for you over the phone that you can pick up at a 24-hour pharmacy. I don't know you, and I don't know your medical history. You could be anybody."

"Well, right now," you tell him, "I think I feel like nobody."

Perhaps he thinks you work for the DEA, the Drug Enforcement Agency, which has been cracking down on pain clinics in Florida. They've been throwing a lot of doctors in jail for turning their prescription pads into money trees.

"What can I do?" you ask. "The pain is killing me."

"Diclofenac," he repeats. He's making some kind of decision. "You got any Advil liquid gels?"

"Yes," you answer.

"You got any extra-strength Tylenol?"

"Yes."

"Take two of the gels and one Tylenol," he says. "And call your doctor in the morning. Who's your primary doctor?"

"Doctor Barish," you answer.

He is silent.

"Who the hell are you?" he suddenly asks. "Doctor Barish hasn't been in the office for over a week."

"I know, but you asked me who my primary doctor was. I am seeing Doctor Abreu while she's away." You are a little angry at his insinuation. "Ah-BREY-You," you repeat, pronouncing the doctor's name correctly.

"Good," he says. "Call him first thing. The office opens at nine-thirty. Good luck."

You head for the medicine cabinet. The concoction makes you feel a little queasy, but some of the pain subsides, not all of it, but at least some of it.

It takes about three hours to get the right prescription sent to Costco on Friday.

It takes another two hours to get it filled.

You take another Advil/Tylenol combination during the waiting period.

Nobody apologizes for the screw-up, but it doesn't matter.

You take your first Diclofenac pill after a light dinner of Kellogg's Special K and strawberries. You eat a little differently when

Kerstin is away; the second choice was blueberry pancakes and sausage. You go to bed early.

The next morning you take another pill. You spend most of Saturday watching television and bringing your real estate websites back to life, but the pain does not go away. You take the third pill in the late afternoon and go to sleep.

It's dark out when the television wakes you up. You roll over, get another pill, swallow it with the water on your bedside table, turn off the TV, and go back to sleep. You do not know if you have pain. All you register is "tired." Maybe a little dizzy, too.

At about 9 a.m. on Sunday, you slowly open your eyes. You feel numb, and you roll over, put your feet on the floor and freeze. Blood blisters cover your entire lower body. They look like leeches, but under the skin, dozens and dozens of them. Your feet have ballooned up at least 30%, and you think they will burst. You stand up. You can hardly walk.

You thump around on two large marshmallows that feel as if they have pins sticking into the bottom of them.

You reach for your iPhone and text Kerstin. It's mid-afternoon in Sweden. Two words. "Come home."

She texts back almost immediately. "I am already on my way."

She knew. Somehow, she knew.

You struggle to sit at a computer in the bedroom. You don't think you can make it up the spiral staircase to your office on the second floor. You type an e-mail to Christan Martone, PA, at Florida Hospital in Celebration, with a copy to Doctor Vipul Patel. The subject line says: **"Temple Williams (Patient: 11-10-1942) URGENT."**

For a few months, I was one of your best robotic prostate removal patients. After the massive infection Doctor Patel discovered and removed, my continence was 100%, six weeks after surgery. I was back to light tennis and a little golf.

I had a slight groin pull on June 21st. It may have had something to do with pushing the erection pump too much. On June 23rd, I got a low-grade fever that rose to 104.5

on the 28th of June. On the 29th of June, I saw my Primary Physician (Dr. Abreau replaced my regular Primary, Dr. Susan Barish. I included his phone number). He prescribed seven days of CIPRO. My urine sample was very brown, but no analysis appears done on it. The fever disappeared, but the groin pain intensified. Walking was impossible.

On July 6, Dr. Abreu prescribed Diclofenac 75 mg for the pain. I take medication for high blood pressure. I had a terrible reaction to Diclofenac, which caused blood spots to spread on my feet and groin area. My blood pressure jumped to 180. I stopped the medication immediately.

I am near the end of the 2nd treatment of Cipro. I still have a slight fever, but it stays below 100 degrees. It has become impossible for me to walk normally.

My urine remains very dark.

I think I may need hospitalization. I do not trust my Primary Physicians, but I do believe in Dr. Patel and in you.

I would like an appointment with you at Florida Hospital immediately (it takes my wife and me a few hours to get up there). We are fully covered through Medicare, long-term care, and personal finances to fix me. Please help.

You sit back and look at the screen. You hit "send." The cat, Truffles, is on your lap, a place she rarely visits on humans. She is not a lap cat, but she's damp. Your tears are falling on the cat. You whisper to Kerstin thousands of miles away, a little amazed: "You knew."

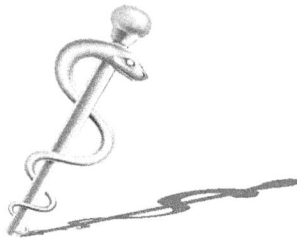

Warrior Patient Rule 6: If you need help, get it. Bravery is for dead people. Pain can be a good thing, a roadmap for doctors, but remember that pain pills hide problems, they do not fix them.

Chapter 7

Hands of Death and Destruction

The 10,623rd best medical school in the world

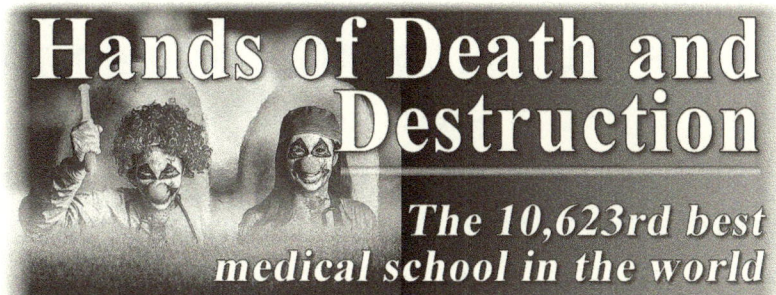

Foreigners, not Swedes, fill the streets of Stockholm on summer weekends. Most of the Swedes disappear into their summer homes.

Their boats sail through the crystal waves of an island-rich Archipelago.

Their laughter mixes with summer songs, drifting across country fields as tourists march up and down the medieval streets of Stockholm's Old Town.

The foreigners visit museums, crowd around the postcard harbor of the city, listen to free concerts in manicured parks. Everything is pretty much closed on summer weekends, especially if the weather is beautiful. Museums, tourist attractions, and restaurants remain open, but many of the stores have handwritten notes on their doors: "stängt för semester." Closed for summer.

An old Cold War joke in the 1970s suggests that a single company of Russian soldiers can successfully invade Sweden if they march on Stockholm in late June or early July.

Kerstin calls Delta Airlines in Stockholm when she gets the Sunday morning text message: "Come home." She gets the same response she would get from most Swedish companies, a rushed young female voice saying: *"Vänligen ring tillbaka när kontoret öppnar på måndag."* Call back when the office opens on Monday, please.

The Swedes have gone to play.

Kerstin needs to cut her trip in half and return to America as quickly as possible.

When the Delta Airlines office opens on Monday, she wants to be sitting on a plane heading over the North Sea. She will fly over Greenland, down the northeastern corridor of Canada and the United States, bound for the Sunshine State of Florida.

She's staying in a guest apartment in the building where a longtime friend lives, Lucie Godber. Lucie is a neighbor in Boca Raton, where she spends her winters with Rocky, a dog who is strangely in love with your cat, HiJinks. Rocky tries to use HiJinks as a soft, chew toy with minimal success. Lucie Godber's son, Eric, is a Delta pilot, but nothing can develop from that. He's impossible to get hold of, and even if it happened, getting Kerstin on a flight would be an unfair and probably impossible task to suggest to him.

The guest apartment where Kerstin is staying is part of the Danvikshem project. The main building is a magnificent, spired brick structure overlooking Stockholm's harbor entrance. It took thirteen years to build at the beginning of the 20th Century. It looks like a more like a castle than an apartment building.

Shortly after the builders mortared the last brick into place in 1915, and the ornate spire rose majestically over the harbor, a visiting military gunboat sailed into Stockholm. The Captain slowed engines in front of Danvikshem, which was and still is a home for the aged. He brought the vessel bristling with guns to "All Stop." As the colossal boat drifted beneath the shadow of Danvikshem's ornate spire, the Captain ordered a full military salute. The cannons of the gunboat boomed out their greeting, shaking the windows and foundation of Danvikshem. The Captain had mistaken the structure for the King's Palace on Gamla Stan, several miles further up the harbor entry to Stockholm. Nobody knows how many elderly residents' lives were cut short by the Gunboat Captain's thunderous, echoing arrival.

Lucie Godber's building is adjacent to Danvikshem, part of the project, with the same magnificent view but a younger crowd. Kerstin's guest quarters have a kitchen, bath, bedroom, and sitting room, but it has no Internet access to help her book a new flight to America.

Kerstin pulls out her cell phone.

The Honorary Consul of Sweden, Per-Olof Lööf, a good friend who lives in Hillsboro, just below Boca Raton, is in Sweden for the summer. He and his wife, Åsa-Lena, are in their car. They have just gotten off the Östanå ferry on the mainland from their summer compound on Ljusterö, an island in the Stockholm archipelago. They're on their way to a summer party — the mobile phone rings in their car, and Åsa-Lena immediately answers.

"Åsa-Lena," Kerstin says, "Temple is sick, badly sick, and I need to get back to America. I need to get on a plane tomorrow morning. The Delta office is closed."

They talk, and Per-Olof will ring back. Right now, he's driving, and the Swedes pay attention to the law about not talking on a mobile phone when you're behind the wheel. He pulls to the side of the road and calls back almost immediately. He gives Kerstin a phone number to the Delta office in London.

Kerstin dials the British number, gets through immediately. Quickly, she gets through to the Delta hub in Paris, France.

She talks to a concerned agent at the Charles De Gaulle airport.

"This is a medical emergency," Kerstin says. "My husband is very sick. He may die."

She receives a business class ticket on a flight from Stockholm to Atlanta, Georgia, first thing Monday morning with a connection from Atlanta to West Palm Beach.

"I'll be at Palm Beach International at 8 PM," she says on the phone.

"I'll meet you there," you say. "I can do that. It's just a thirty-minute trip. We will drive up to Florida Hospital Celebration first thing on Tuesday."

On Monday morning, as Kerstin is pushed back in her seat on takeoff from Arlanda Airport outside Stockholm, you are watching a bad movie about vampires and walking dead people on television in Boca Raton. The clock flashes green on the cable box: "2:34 am." You push the off button on the remote control. The television turns black.

You finally fall asleep. You have put an extra sheet on your side of the bed in case any of the blood blisters pop.

When you wake up in the morning, you search for a set of shoes into which you can cram your feet. You find an old, oversized pair of sneakers in the back of the closet, remove the laces and shoehorn the marshmallows below your ankles into them. Your skin tears at the back of your left foot, leaving an open wound. The right foot makes it into the laceless sneakers without any bloodletting.

You stomp your way out to the car, a little surprised at how well you can move and drive to Personal Physicians Associates. It's early, and only three patients are waiting for their appointments. A technician comes out and turns on the TV that nobody watches.

"May I help you?" the receptionist asks. She takes her eyes off the appointment pad and looks up when you do not answer immediately.

"I need to see Doctor Abreu," you say. "I do not have an appointment." She stares at you and starts to open her mouth. You lean into the window a bit. "I do have blood blisters all over my groin and legs from the prescription that Doctor Abreu gave me on Friday, and I need to see him. Now."

"Your name?" she asks. You answer: "Temple Williams ... eleven, ten, forty-two."

Your birth date. More important than your first and last name.

She writes this down, taps her computer keyboard, lifts the phone, and speaks to someone, probably the doctor's assistant.

"Take a seat," she says. "The doctor will be right with you."

Fifteen minutes later, you follow a nurse into an examination room. The nurse assistant walks quickly ahead of you, down the hallway, then slows and stops as she turns and sees you struggling far behind her.

They don't weigh you; they don't take your blood pressure. Doctor Abreu enters, concerned, in a nicely starched white doctor's jacket with his stethoscope around his neck.

"I had a pretty bad reaction to the medication you put me on," you say. "You know, the one it took you a couple of days to get right at the prescription desk at Costco?"

"It's the computer system," he says. "It's new. Sorry." He finally looks at you. "The nurse said you had some blisters?"

You pull down your pants.

You show him your blood blisters from your groin to your feet. You turn your left foot and show him the open wound on your ankle, surrounded by dried blood.

"Wow," he says.

"Wow," you repeat, slowly. "Tell me, is that a professional medical opinion?" You pull up your pants and hitch your belt. He looks at you, tries to smile a little, but realizes you are angry. His mouth shifts into neutral.

He sits down, taps on a black keyboard. "I guess that's not the right prescription," he says to the computer screen. There is a moment of absolute silence. Then you burst out laughing. It startles you as well as him. He does not know if he can trust your apparent good humor. You look around the office for some blunt instrument with which you can beat him to death.

There is a commotion outside the examination room. Someone opens the door and asks for Doctor Abreu to come out. He escapes quickly, and the door closes, but not completely. You open the door some more and watch Doctor Abreu in a lively discussion with a large angry man at the end of the hall. A small, rectangular woman stands slightly to the right of the men. She could easily be a puppet, half the size of the person with her. You think the angry man is her husband, but possibly her son; she seems much older than him. The woman looks like an old cereal box in a faded multi-colored dress, with two legs, a head and arms sticking out of it.

The large man's voice fills the corridor.

"God damned it," he says, pronouncing each word precisely. "She walks like a duck, she talks like a duck, she acts like a duck, and all you give me are some frigging pills to fix her! You need to FIX her!" His face is bright red with resentment and anger.

The poor woman waddles around in a circle to prove the man's point, a small desperate dance that seems both tragic and comical.

The big man is shaking an orange container of pills in Doctor Abreu's face. Doctor Abreu tries to calm him down, in a voice so low you cannot hear what is said. The big man's shoulders slump. Doctor Abreu puts his hand on the woman's shoulder. She has stopped dancing. The big man shakes his head back and forth, seemingly beaten by Doctor Abreu's words. He turns and walks away. The woman waddles behind him.

Every year, according to the Reuters news wire, 100,000 patients are killed, and nine million hurt in the United States because of medical mistakes. There is a deadly ghost drifting on the frayed edges of the medical world. His name is Doctor Hodad.

Most second-year medical students have heard about Doctor Hodad, an acronym for Hands Of Death And Destruction. There are many Doctor Hodads in the hospitals, clinics, treatment, and health centers of America.

A leading surgeon at Johns Hopkins, Doctor Marty Makary, writes a book about it: *Unaccountable: What Hospitals Won't Tell You and How Transparency Can Revolutionize Health Care.* He meets his Doctor Hodad as a medical student at the Boston hospital, where he receives training.

Doctor Makary explains in his book: "He was one of the surgeons most requested by patients, including celebrities, thanks to his charming bedside manner and their lack of understanding about what caused their post-op problems." This Hodad has an unfortunate tendency to screw up operations badly. His mistakes suffer life-threatening complications.

Sadly there is little, often no accountability in medicine. Like it or not, accept it or not, if physicians are not legally bound to report something, they won't. When they participate in surveys measuring patient care or safety, they always do so under the condition that the results remain a secret from the public.

Of course, some transparency does exist in the medical world, but it remains an exception and not a rule, with no real or substantial guidelines. Doctor Marty Makary, now famous as the man who dragged Doctor Hodad out of the closet, writes an excellent article in The Wall Street Journal on September 21, 2012. In that article, he points out that if medical errors were a disease, they would be the sixth leading cause of death in America. The first two paragraphs of his article warrant repeating:

When there is a plane crash in the U.S., even a minor one, it makes headlines. There is a thorough federal investigation, and the tragedy often yields important lessons for the aviation industry. Pilots and airlines thus learn how to do their jobs more safely.

The world of American medicine is far deadlier: Medical mistakes kill enough people each week to fill four jumbo jets. But these mistakes go largely unnoticed by the world at large, and the medical community rarely learns from them. The same preventable mistakes are made over and over again, and patients are left in the dark about which hospitals have significantly better (or worse) safety records than their peers.

Pill-pushing Doctors qualify as Hodads-in-training. Primary Physicians throw a prescription in a patient's hand and hope for the best.

Often it works.

The number of sick and older people squeezing into America's health care system makes pill-pushing a natural approach to wellness, a financial path of least resistance.

"Take two aspirin and call me in the morning," turns from a tired joke into a questionable and often dangerous medical approach because the pills in your hand are no longer just aspirin.

Now they are pharmaceutical wonder drugs that many doctors issue inappropriately. They receive little or no training to know who should, or should not swallow the pill. And some of the doctors are just plain stupid.

The prescription Doctor Abreu gives you, Diclofenac, is a nonsteroidal anti-inflammatory drug that relieves pain, swelling, and joint stiffness caused by arthritis. Arthritis, as far as you can tell, is not a problem for you.

Diclofenac is not suitable for people with high blood pressure (hypertension), which most definitely is a problem for you. Your medical information, available online at Personal Physician Care, where Doctor Abreu works, clearly notes this. Doctor Barish, your primary doctor, who is currently in Europe with her family, has you on a daily dose of 12.5mg of Losartan. It is a drug used almost exclusively for high blood pressure, a medical diagnosis from which you suffer.

Diclofenac can cause drowsiness and dizziness. Your dosage is one tablet every 12 hours. You get through 4 tablets in two days before blood blisters cover the lower half of your body, with an open wound on your heel.

The merry-go-round of pill-pushing leaves money in a doctor's pocket. He or she gets paid, moves on. If the medical situation deteriorates into a more difficult problem, the doctor refers the patient to a specialist. Order some expensive and often unnecessary tests first. The primary doctor moves the patient along the medical yellow brick road, doing nothing wrong.

"I guess that's not the right prescription."

Next patient.

Since meeting Doctor Abreu a week earlier, you have researched his background thoroughly. You do not discover one single thing that makes you comfortable with his advice or his medical knowledge.

He graduates from medical school in 1993, in Havana, Cuba. His school is called Instituto Superior De Ciencias Medicas De La Habana. In English, this means "Higher Institute of Medical Sciences of Havana."

You know that most, but not all, graduates of Caribbean Medical Schools, who work as doctors after moving to the United States, attend those institutions because they fail to meet the higher entry requirements of their counterparts in the United States.

The Higher Institute of Medical Sciences of Havana opens its doors in 1976. It is considered the 15th best medical school in Cuba, according to the Education Database on the popular ranking website, Classbase.

The Higher Institute of Medical Sciences of Havana ranks as the 705th best medical school in Latin America.

The Higher Institute of Medical Sciences of Havana ranks as the 10,623rd best medical school in the world.

Being the patient of a doctor who graduates from the 10,623rd best medical school in the world is not something about which you want to brag.

When Doctor Abreu returns to the examination room after he meets with the large man and small woman in the corridor, he apologizes for the delay.

He starts tapping the keyboard of his medical information computer.

"What to do," he says to the computer screen. "What to do."

"I know what to do," you say.

He stops typing and looks at you.

You stand up, walk slowly and carefully out of the examination room, painfully through the waiting room, out to the parking lot, into your car, and back to the safety of your home.

Within a year, Doctor Abreau will be arrested and thrown in jail. His bond will be half a million dollars.

In ten more hours, Kerstin's Delta flight will touch down at Palm Beach International Airport.

You check to see if there is any response from the e-mail you have sent to Christan

Martone, PA, at the Florida Hospital Celebration. There is none.

You sit down and write, on a yellow legal pad, what you want to say to her, then realize that it is all in the e-mail. You are not thinking clearly. You dial the number of the Global Robotics Institute, and after a few minutes, Christan comes on the line.

Before she can say anything, you blurt out what you have written in the e-mail, stopping for air just four times.

You add that Kerstin is returning from Europe as you speak, that she will arrive around eight o'clock in the evening, and that you can drive up early the next morning.

There is silence. Christan wants to make sure you fully vent.

"I just read your e-mail," Christan says in a soft voice. "Of course, we will take care of you. We will be here waiting for you, and we will take care of you."

"Thank you," you say. "Thank you."

You hang up the phone. Relief washes over you. You sob like a small child.

You embarrass yourself, but you cannot stop for several minutes.

Kerstin's plane touches down on time. She has already cleared customs in Atlanta. She sees you sitting in the baggage area.

You don't get up to hug her because you do not think you can stand up very straight. It does not take long before you struggle back to the car in short-term parking. She gets behind the wheel and drives you back home. When she sees your blood blisters and the open wound on your left foot, she is horrified.

You sleep, get up, and leave for Florida Hospital before six o'clock. At 9:15, you drive up to the hospital in Celebration and meet Christan Martone, PA.

Your previous stay at the Florida Hospital has been for one night.

This time, it will last 13 days, and you will discover that the number "13" deserves its reputation for bad luck.

Life is about to change, perhaps forever.

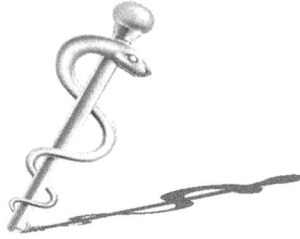

<u>Warrior Patient Rule 7</u>: Doctors who go to excellent medical schools are better than doctors who go to poorly-rated medical schools. There are no exceptions to this, NONE.

Chapter 8

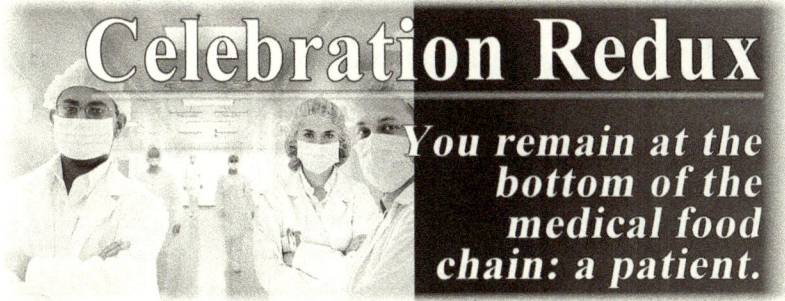

Celebration Redux

You remain at the bottom of the medical food chain: a patient.

"We're taking him right to the emergency room," Christan Martone says to Kerstin as you pull up Florida Hospital Celebration.

"I don't feel that bad," you say, immediately realizing how foolish that must sound under the circumstances.

"The emergency room," Christan repeats. The order, she points out, has come directly from Doctor Vipul Patel.

They take a blood test and a CT (Computed Tomography) scan on your abdomen and pelvis. CT scanning is a painless X-Ray procedure that peeks into your body in a series of cross-sectional slices of soft tissue, bone, and blood vessels. The process has advanced enormously since its first use in 1974.

After the scan, they hook you up to an IV, install a catheter, and move you into a room with a view on the third floor, Room 351. You're mildly offended by the catheterization. You have worked hard to kick diapers out of your life. Thousands of Kegel exercises guarantee that you will be drier than a Pamper on the floor of Death Valley. But you also know that nurses prefer patients who are bagged and tagged. They are less trouble. You can avoid them for hours.

Kerstin stays with you into the evening, with a short break in the afternoon to check into the hotel where she stayed when you had your radical prostatectomy.

Doctor Patel visits and tells you that they will get to the bottom of this and have you up and going as quickly as possible.

"I was doing great," you tell him. "Totally continent within five weeks." You pull back the sheet and lift your leg, hoping he'll order the catheter removed. He nods, and he knows you don't need it. But it stays.

"We will get to the bottom of this," he repeats. You smile, consider making a stupid remark about how urologists always get to the bottom of things, since that is their theater of operations. You resist. Doctor Patel is not the sort of person with whom you joke around.

"Thank you," you finally say. "You are a great doctor." He nods slightly and leaves.

The blood blisters start to fade fairly quickly. The wound on your foot takes longer. Within a few days, thewy diagnose you with normocytic anemia, leukocytosis, and thrombocytosis. All of this sounds dangerous, and it is, but it's not life-threatening. You test negative for malignant cells, so there's no new cancer playing pinball with your body parts.

Normocytic anemia often occurs in men and women over 85 years old. At the time, you are almost 70 and look and feel younger. Your red blood cells are getting whacked. These are the guys that take oxygen to all the essential parts of your body. Your red blood cells are normal-sized, but you are not producing enough of them. It can happen for a lot of reasons.

"I think they immediately ruled out pregnancy," you tell Kerstin much later. She gives you a lopsided grin and bears it.

There are two kinds of normocytic anemia, congenital (you're born with it) and acquired (you catch it). You appear to have acquired normocytic anemia, often associated with infection. You wake in the morning feeling worn out. You remain worn out throughout the day. You got to sleep feeling worn out.

The most common cause of acquired normocytic anemia is a long-term (chronic) disease. It can be cancer, arthritis, or kidney disease. Some medicines can also cause you to have normocytic anemia, but this does not happen often.

You do not know if what Doctor Abreu gave you, Diclofenac, is a suspect.

You need to understand a significant "Warrior Patient" point at this stage. As this book unfolds, the patient might sound pretty smart about a lot of things. But in reality, you know almost nothing. Doctors and nurses tell you almost nothing. You remain in the dark about virtually everything. You do not know what questions to ask, or what answers to expect.

You are the lowest animal in the medical food chain. You are a patient.

The diagnosis of leukocytosis includes something called "an absolute neutrophilic left shift." It is not a dance step, but it's relatively common. What it means is that your white blood cell count jumps above its normal range. The left shift means that the ratio of immature to mature white cells increases, mostly due to infection.

"Again," you tell Kerstin much later, "I think they immediately ruled out pregnancy."

"Drop the baby," she warns.

"That's cold," you say, but you get it.

Thrombocytosis means you have a high platelet count in your blood. Platelets are blood cells whose function is to stop the bleeding. Only mammals have platelets, an adaptation that probably evolves to offset the risk of bleeding at childbirth (unique to mammals).

"In other words," you tell Kerstin much later (she narrows her eyes expecting another pregnancy test), " ... I clot easily." It becomes significant in another month, although you have no idea what "thrombocytosis" means at the time. You don't even know you have it.

Two days after arriving at Florida Hospital, Dawn Bowles, a nurse working there, gives you a renal (kidney) ultrasound exam.

She smears translucent paste over your lower back and swirls it around slowly with a monitoring device. Both the left and the right kidney appear healthy, with no mass and no urine buildup, no swelling (they empty fine into the bladder), and no kidney stones. It seems that the kidneys work fine.

None of this would have been too challenging to explain upfront. Doctors and nurses treat you with dignity and warmth, and they treat Kerstin with broad smiles and friendship as she spends her days with you. But they do not reveal anything.

Doctors often hide silently behind a mask of science. It's easier that way.

"Nothing can slow down the medical process faster than a patient who knows just enough to be dangerous." Concealment remains a prevailing attitude in hospitals and clinics throughout America.

Kerstin returns to Boca Raton for a few days, and you continue to mend in your comfortable room at the hospital in Celebration. Doctors come and go, poke and prod, laugh, and enjoy your smiling wisecracks. Well, not always.

One night, late, a handsome doctor you have never seen before comes into your dimly lit room, trailing an attractive young internist in his wake. From her exotic accent, as she talks to him in a hushed voice, she appears to be a Brazilian beauty. You spend time in Mozambique, Africa, in the mid-1960s, with Frelimo's Freedom Fighters, and you know a female Portuguese accent when you hear one. The good-looking doctor is making his rounds. You are playing dead (which is probably not a smart thing to do in a hospital, although it works this time).

The doctor you never met leans into the internist and whispers about you as if you're a piece of meat, an old piece of meat. You have never seen this physician before, but you know that his "hands-on" approach to medicine will have little to do with the patient he is visiting. The internist appears very young and innocent.

You lift your head and look at him, and they are both startled that you are awake. You hitch your index finger at the Portuguese beauty. She leans close. You say, loud enough for him to hear: "He has a wife and seven kids, and he makes women have babies just by looking at them. *Porquino*." The last is a nickname, in Portuguese, for one of the men you taught to blow stuff up in Africa: "Little Pig."

She jerks her head up at the good-looking doctor. He jerks his thumb towards the door, signaling that this patient's visit is over. You never see either of them again.

"Maybe it was a dream," Kerstin tells you when she returns on the weekend.

You lower your reading glasses and drop your chin. "Maybe it wasn't," you say. "What bothered me the most was the way he was whispering about me like a piece of old meat and how difficult he told her it was to find a solution to my problems. I never saw this doctor before in my life."

Much later, you tell this story to your good friend Brian Greenman as you sit under an umbrella on tennis court #2 where he lives. He speaks Portuguese, having spent much of his youth in Brazil. He understands *"Porquino"* and laughs at the story. He feels sorry for a man with such a nickname.

You are playing singles, and you're ahead four to three, but you're still on serve. Rain is in the process of washing out the game.

Most people Brian's age slump in wheelchairs or push walkers, but he is thin and trim, and he chases after tennis balls like a teenager. When you play doubles, Kerstin wants him as her partner, not you.

Brian stops running six miles a day when he is in his eighties. Everyone has to slow down a little. He still jumps rope. With the hard rain almost drowning out his words under the umbrella, he tells me a story about older people in hospitals.

"I used to know a doctor in New York, still do know him, and they have a nickname for old patients in the hospital where he works: they called them 'Lox.' You know, salmon. They would sneer, oh, there's a Lox in room 403. I gotta go see a Lox in Room 227."

Back at Florida Hospital in Celebration, you remind Kerstin that patients are the lowest animal in the medical food chain.

"Lower than lab rats?" she asks you. She nails you again. "Patients are most certainly a lab rat's equal," I admit.

She smiles at you and runs her hand up your leg as you lie in bed. "Don't get any funny ideas," you say to her.

"Your skin is very tight and smooth," she says. "It's amazing." The blood blisters have entirely disappeared. The open wound on the back of your left foot has almost healed. The pain goes away completely.

You have a severe infection, and the reason your skin is so tight and smooth is that the doctors are pumping a lot of antibiotics and infection-fighting drugs into you.

You are bloated, huge.

You struggle out of bed and stumble into the bathroom.

You recognize the man you see in the mirror, but only from the neck up. The doctors and nurses manage to attach a whole new body to your head.

In a little over a week, they add an extra 30 pounds to your frame. You look like you're auditioning for the longest-running show on Broadway, New York's Macy's Thanksgiving Day Balloon Parade.

On your seventh day in the hospital, you go for a second CT scan of your abdomen and pelvis. The left-side muscles in your lower back are enlarged and inflamed, and the soft tissue density around them shows abnormalities.

The swelling could be the result of a hematoma from the fall on the tennis court a year earlier when blood leaks into the muscle with nowhere to go. Your body puts an envelope on it, isolating it, water in a balloon.

The CT scan also detects Diverticulosis, probably related to the adjacent inflammation. It's a problem in the colon that can be painful, but you have a very mild case. You do not suffer from it at all. You don't even know you have it.

The CT scan also detects hernias. No pop-up has yet appeared in your abdomen, but it will. The hernias, you believe, are the offspring of the penis pump. The tissue has torn, muscles weakened, in your attempts to set Willie free.

"How do you feel?" Kerstin asks you after the new CT scan.

"Very large," you say. "I am gaining weight every day."

"I was walking past the nurses' station," Kerstin says, "and a doctor was there shaking her head at the computer screen. I talked to her. She says she just doesn't know what's causing all your problems. She's very frustrated."

"Well, if they don't figure it out pretty soon, I'm going to blow up like the glutton in that Monty Python film," you tell Kerstin.

It is a funny skit. A hugely fat man gorges himself in a fancy restaurant, ordering food and insulting waiters. Suddenly he bursts like a balloon filled with body parts and spaghetti. All that's left is a swollen, empty rib cage beneath his flapping jowls.

He has a surprised look on his face.

It doesn't seem all that funny anymore.

After the first week, Doctor Patel has lost interest in you. He still directs your care, but in his opinion, your problem has nothing to do with the radical prostatectomy performed a few months earlier. He has a huge business to run, and it will not operate without him. The robot needs Doctor Patel.

The doctor you see the most while you are at Florida Hospital Celebration is Doctor Divya K. Navani, specializing in internal medicine and a Hospitalist.

The term Hospitalist means she is a case manager, sort of a temporary Primary Doctor for hospitalized patients. They coordinate medications and diagnostic tests. They visit you on their rounds a couple of times every day. Doctor Navani has a soft face and a quick smile, and she's stunning and easily amused by your humor. She has been a medical doctor for over 18 years.

Another doctor is now involved in your case, Doctor Praneetha Puskuri, the doctor that is shaking her head at the computer screen when

Kerstin arrives. Although you do not know it at the time, nor do you know what it means, she is a Nephrologist, a kidney doctor. She does not work at the Florida Hospital Celebration. You do not see her that often.

Doctor Puskuri is one of eight doctors at the Heart of Florida Regional Medical Center, who specializes in Nephrology. She travels a lot. She is licensed in New Jersey, where her primary practice seems to exist, as well as in Texas and Florida. She has been a Nephrologist for many years, and she is good at it.

She has a Fellowship in Nephrology at the Albert Einstein College of Medicine from 2008 to 2010.

You know none of this at the time, only that she is a lovely doctor who appears genuinely concerned about you.

But the knowledge of how or why she is there, doctoring you, remains a secret. You assume she works for Doctor Patel. She does not. You believe she is part of the Global Robotics Institute of Florida Hospital in Celebration. She is not.

Once again, you remain at the bottom of the medical food chain: a patient. A veil of secrecy keeps knowledge of what is going on well beyond your reach, and well beyond the grasp of Kerstin.

"You know," you tell Kerstin much later, "specialization is a double-edged sword. Well, maybe double-edged scalpel is a better analogy."

"What are you talking about?"

"A specialist sees you as his or her specialty," you say. "But he or she doesn't connect the dots to all your other problems."

"That's not their job," Kerstin says.

"*Do no harm* is their job," you answer. "That's the oath. But a prostate surgeon views me as a prostate. A kidney surgeon views me as a kidney. An infectious diseases doctor views me like an infection."

"That's a bad thing?" she asks.

"No," you admit. "I guess that's necessary. But it can also put blinkers on the specialists, narrowing their focus dangerously. Pointing them in just one direction. They need to see the whole picture of a patient to be great doctors."

Kerstin thinks about this for a moment. Then she says: "That's what good primary doctors are for." She thinks she knows her stuff.

"Good luck with that," you answer. You know the reality. It takes you months to discover nurse practitioners, the glue that brings patient care into a proper perspective.

Even before that, within a month, you will meet a truly great doctor.

But right now, at the Global Robotics Institute of Florida Hospital in Celebration, Doctor Praneetha Puskuri has her medical crosshairs pointing at an abscess at the bottom of the hematoma in your back.

She orders a CT-guided left pelvic fluid collection. They're going to punch a needle into you and drain the abscess.

Nurses wheel you down to the radiology department, where you meet a nice guy with a huge needle. Doctor Nicholas Feranec has been a radiologist for a decade, educated at the University of Florida College of Medicine. He practices at Florida Hospital in Celebration as well as further north in Gainesville.

You tell him about induction day at Parris Island, South Carolina, when you joined the Marine Corps in 1961. The big needle gets you into this subject.

"They lined up all the recruits and marched us through the barracks. They inoculated us with a bunch of different vaccines. There were corpsmen on either side of us with metal-air guns punching holes in our arms," you tell the radiologist.

Pop. Pop. Step forward, recruit. Pop. Pop. Then out the back door of the barracks with trickles of blood running down your arms.

"Love it," Doctor Feranec says.

"You need to lie on your back on the CT table," his assisting nurse tells you. "Can you make it by yourself?"

"Like a beached whale," you answer, conscious of your newly-acquired girth.

"So anyway," you continue, "our Drill Instructor is standing just inside the barracks door, and when a particularly tough-acting recruit steps inside, the Drill Instructor holds up a Bible."

"A Bible," the Doctor repeats.

"Yup. And he tells the recruit to put the Bible under his arm so the needle won't go all the way through. The big tough guy faints."

The Doctor and nurse laugh politely. They've probably heard it before. The doctor turns to the nurse: "Do we have the Old Testament handy?" he asks.

"I prefer the King James' version," you say. The laughter is a little harder; yourself included. Everyone is having fun.

The doctor numbs you with 1% lidocaine and then goes into the abscess at the bottom of the hematoma near the kidney and drains it. The needle sucks up 25 mL of pus.

Given its deep location and small size, they do not place a drain in the abscess. The fluid will be cultured and examined. A sterile dressing is applied.

It is all over in 20 minutes, with no problem. An assistant wheels you back to your charming room with a view.

Later in the afternoon, you return for a CT-guided right kidney biopsy. This time you are on your stomach. The needle looks bigger. You are too tired to joke around.

The CT scan takes images of your kidneys. They prep your right flank and drape it in sterile surgical fashion. The doctor numbs you with twice as much lidocaine as the earlier drainage procedure. They position a 17 gauge biopsy system over your right kidney. Next, they perform two 18 gauge core biopsies on the kidney. Chunk, chunk. You don't feel a thing. Sterile dressing. Twenty minutes. An assistant wheels ou back to your room.

Twenty-four hours later, you get another CT scan of your abdomen and pelvis. They need to check the result of the biopsy and the drainage, and they need to make sure there is no internal bleeding.

There is a minor thickening of the left wall of the bladder. If the doctor had asked you about it, you could have told him that this was probably the result of distending your bladder during the Great Catheter Wars, which followed the original prostate biopsy.

They do not ask.

You remain at the bottom of the medical food chain.

The pocket of infection that they drained yesterday has already filled up again. But no new hematoma, although some muscle inflammation continues.

"So now I have a new Doctor on the team trying to save me," you tell Kerstin.

"Who is he?" she asks.

"Doctor Siddiqui," you answer, and on cue, he enters the room. He's a very dignified man. Put him in a police lineup, and he's the one you pick as "the doctor."

Doctor Shoaib Anwer Siddiqui's specialty is infectious diseases. He works for Florida Hospital Celebration.

"We have analyzed the fluid drained from you," he tells us. "As I suspected when I talked to you before, the fluid is positive for MRSA." He does not say the letters. He says, "Mersa."

"Is that bad?" Kerstin asks.

"It is not good. But we will treat it."

"Can you beat it?" she asks.

"We will treat it," he repeats.

After he walks out of the room, you notice that the air quality has deteriorated quite a bit. "Boy," you say, "I guess he likes Indian food." Pungent aromas from an Indian Restaurant spice the air.

"Mersa does not sound good," Kerstin tells you without a smile.

"We can fight it," you tell her. "We can fight anything."

MRSA is an acronym for Methicillin-resistant Staphylococcus aureus, a dangerous infection caused by a strain of staph bacteria.

It remains resistant to antibiotics usually used to treat ordinary staph infections.

Most MRSA infections occur in hospitals, clinics, and healthcare settings, although a new strain has started to occur among healthy people, where it often starts as a painful skin boil.

MRSA can burrow deep into the body, causing life-threatening infections in bones, joints, surgical wounds, the heart valves, the kidneys, the lungs, the prostate.

My mind wanders back to where everything started.

"I wonder why you're so infected?" Doctor Gottenger asks, but he never answers the question.

He never tries.

Doctor Patel locks his eyes on you after you mention to him that you still feel a little infected a week after the radical prostatectomy.

"The infection is no longer there," he says. "It is gone."

But it is not. It is waiting. And now its hiding place has been discovered.

They treat MRSA with super drugs, antibiotics that overpower a staph infection that resists standard treatment.

Vancomycin is the silver bullet of choice. People who go through the process call it "getting vanked." An IV pouch of Vancomycin hangs above you and slowly drips the clear liquid into your bloodstream. It can take more than an hour to empty the bag.

As you approach your final days at the Florida Hospital Celebration, you weigh almost 260 pounds (your average weight is around 195), and you are on six different medications.

Amlodipine is a calcium channel blocker that widens blood vessels and improves blood flow. It treats high blood pressure.

Colace is a stool softener.

Lasix is a diuretic that wrings the excess water out of your body, although it doesn't seem to work very well.

You are a bloated balloon.

Labetalol is another medication used to treat high blood pressure.

"It often treats hypertension during pregnancy," you tell Kerstin.

"Stop it," she says.

"As long as I'm here with all these wonderful doctors," you say, "maybe I should have a sex change."

She laughs, and you stop. You get it.

The fifth medication in your arsenal of medical weapons is Pantoprazole, which sounds like something on an Italian menu.

It's for heartburn, which most Italian cuisines deliver free of charge.

You don't even know that you suffer from heartburn.

The final medication is Vancomycin. They constantly drip bags of "Vanc" into your body through an IV. The super drug will destroy the MRSA infection., but there is a delicate balancing act involved in it. Vancomycin requires cautious use in patients who suffer from reduced kidney function.

A company in Arkansas named Nephropath analyzes your kidney biopsy. It turns out that somebody has whacked your kidneys. The small blood vessels in the tissue sample submitted have moderate to severe Arteriosclerosis and Arteriolosclerosis, a hardening and loss of elasticity of the walls of both the large and the small arteries. The tissue surrounding the arteries is inflamed. And MRSA appears to be the culprit. The report concludes that the presence of the inflammation "raises suspicion of interstitial nephritis associated with drug sensitivity." In other words, your kidney disease might be a reaction to a medication.

Two days before you leave Florida Hospital Celebration, a group of doctors gets together to discuss your case. Doctor Padma K.

Raju, a cardiologist at the Osceola Regional Medical Center, calls together the group to discuss a transesophageal echocardiogram. You have no idea what this is, although research much later explains that it is a costly procedure that uses sound waves to create high-quality moving pictures of the heart and its blood vessels.

The average cost is about $4,000, and it can be as high as $11,700.

Doctor Praneetha Puskuri, the kidney doctor, and Doctor Shoaib Anwer Siddiqui, the infectious diseases doctor, are not invited to this meeting.

Doctor Patel attends, and so does Doctor Divya K. Navani, the attractive Hospitalist.

You have no idea who Doctor Padma K. Raju is.

You never meet this doctor.

The consult approves the echocardiogram.

You are vaguely aware that there is a battle, a turf war going on among all the doctors concerning you. Perhaps someone finally said: "Enough. Let him go. Enough."

You never have the expensive (and probably pointless) cardio procedure. You never know about it until long after you never have it. Only the hospital records talk about it, revealed during research for "Warrior Patient."

You are now in your last days at Florida Hospital Celebration. Your final physical says you are well-developed and not in acute distress. You are well-nourished (you're telling me).

Your blood pressure is high, 167/61, and your pulse rate registers 60 beats per minute (you have always had a low pulse). The heart sounds are normal. The lungs have diminished air entry over both bases (guess who's put on 50 pounds). The abdomen is considered "soft" (but you swear there's a six-pack down in there somewhere).

You can stand up and walk, albeit slowly. The terrible pain that brought you to the hospital has completely disappeared.

You have hypertension (high blood pressure) and renal insufficiency (questionable kidneys), although nobody tells you about the kidney thing.

"You saved my life by bringing me here," you tell Kerstin. She dismisses this, but you mean it. "You saved my life." You can hug her standing up, and there's a lot of you to embrace. You are often "vanked."

One more procedure remains before you can go home.

You need a chest PICC ("pick") line so you can continue fighting your infection, getting Vancomycin with a home care nurse. PICC is an acronym for Peripherally Inserted Central Catheter. The world of medicine has too many syllables in it.

A PICC line is a long, thin, flexible tube used to give medicines, like Vancomycin, for weeks or months. The catheter will snake from your inside elbow area, through a vein until it reaches a larger vein near your heart. The procedure does not require a doctor. A nurse with the tongue-twisting designation of the American Registry of Radiologic Technicians (ARRT) and her assistant place the PICC in your arm. Then they X-Ray it with a portable machine to make sure its placement is medically sound.

They are very proud of their miniature X-Ray machine.

Kerstin does not need to watch this, so she leaves to pay the bill, pick up prescriptions at the pharmacy, and get the car ready for our departure. They will wheelchair you downstairs, and you can meet out front.

"Whoops," the PICC-line nurse says, viewing the first X-Ray result. The PICC line has burrowed down to your right hand instead of up to your heart. You have a scar on your right arm from your childhood. You didn't want to take a bath as a five-year-old, and you ran through a plate-glass door to escape outside, getting 19 stitches and a peak preview of your arm's muscle structure. The scar tissue has sent the PICC line in the wrong direction.

"Try the other arm," you say, explaining the problem.

"You must have been a cute kid," the nurse says.

"Well, I was being taken care of by an Irish babysitter with ruby-red lips, and after I had returned from the hospital, she kissed me on the forehead. So it was worth it. I didn't wash the lipstick off for days." We laugh. We're having a good time.

On the left arm, the PICC line reaches for your heart with no problem. You are finally good to go.

The Hospitalist, Doctor Divya K. Navani, has come to say goodbye. She stands by the window and smiles as the nurses leave with their equipment. "I will miss your smile," she says. Her voice trembles and you see that she is crying. "Oh," she says, "You have been through so much." You have a friendship hug, two pats on the back.

"I'll be all right," you say, surprised and humbled by her emotions. In the car heading back to Boca, you tell Kerstin about this parting scene.

"She was crying." You sit and think for a while. "You know what scares me?"

"What?"

"I think maybe she was looking down the path of my future, and all she saw was horrible stuff."

"You're going to be fine," Kerstin says.

You fall asleep in the car, thinking that Doctor Navani saw your future, and she was afraid of it.

You don't know at the time, but she has good reason to cry.

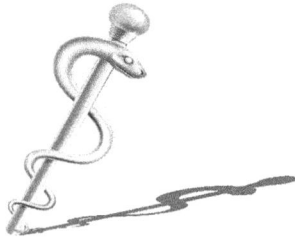

Warrior Patient Rule 8: Try to understand any tests and procedures your doctors suggest. Many just pay for new hospital equipment. Even good doctors enjoy playing with expensive toys. They get paid well for doing it, too.

Chapter 9

Emergency Fever

You spend two days not talking about kidney dialysis. Maybe it will go away.

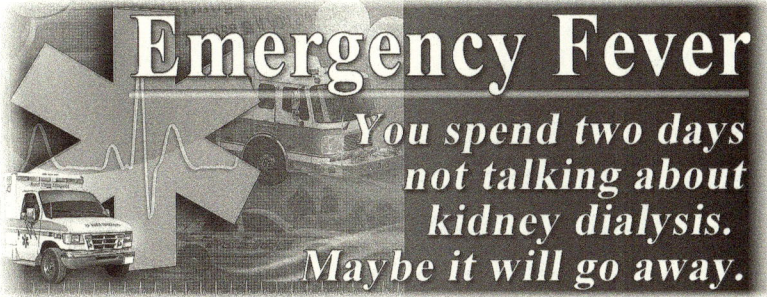

You get home late, and you flop onto a bed that creaks more than usual under new, more substantial management. You have a home-care nurse coming in the morning from an agency called First Stat, although their logo slurs it into a single word: Firstat.

It's part of Ambient Healthcare, Inc., an agency that serves chemical cocktails in the comfort of patients' homes throughout the southeastern United States.

At nine o'clock in the morning, a lovely nurse named Sharonda Shaw shows up. She has Vancomycin, heparin flush, sodium chloride, alcohol prep pads, dressings, vinyl gloves, a quest lab kit, and a portable medicine pole. She hands you a 38-page patient handbook slipped into a folder covered with 36 tightly spaced paragraphs, all with bullet points, outlining a patient's rights and obligations.

"I wonder if anyone ever reads all that stuff," Kerstin asks.

"Only in a court of law," you reply, grinning at Sharonda. She makes sure you're taking your medication: a blood pressure pill, a diuretic that squeezes the excess fluid out of your body, and a pill that improves your blood flow. Sharonda opens boxes of medical stuff and sets up the medicine pole. Doctor Siddiqui, infectious diseases, arranges all this before you ever leave the Florida Hospital three-and-a-half hours north of Boca Raton.

Sharonda draws blood through your new PICC line, sterilizing everything carefully as you sit in your living room watching TV. She takes your blood pressure and pulse, and she hangs a bag of Vancomycin above you on the portable medicine pole. Gravity drains the powerful antibiotic slowly into your heart, through your new PICC line. You like this much better than room 351 at Florida Hospital Celebration. Bigger room. Better television. More channels. And you have fresh snacks from the kitchen.

The home care treatment takes about an hour. Sharonda packs up quickly, careful with the small vials of blood that she'll hand in for analysis. They're essential and necessary, the benchmark they use to determine whether or not you need to go to the hospital.

The next day, a different nurse shows up, and she's in a hurry.

When she pulls into the garage drive, her left rear tire is flat. She has no spare. She's a little angry and frustrated. "My boyfriend is coming to fix it," she says, and he does. She draws your blood, takes your blood pressure, pulse, and temperature, all normal. You get "vanked." Then she leaves.

Kerstin has been playing tennis, and when she returns, she notices something on a glass table between two comfortable chairs in front of the television (you have fallen sound asleep in one of them).

"Oh, my God!" Kerstin shouts, suddenly jarring you awake.

You focus on the TV, expecting some disaster to fill the screen. A large person in a chef's apron cooks spaghetti with lamb meatballs. Meanwhile, Kerstin points at the glass table. Two red vials of your blood are left behind, forgotten.

She calls the phone number on a Firstat business card that says, Lisa Nicely, RN. Lisa tells her, nicely, to refrigerate the blood; someone will retrieve it the following day. You wonder if that's her real name.

"Refrigerate it. No problem."

About 30 hours later, you receive an urgent call from the Delray Hospital telling you to get to the emergency room immediately. Don't delay. Move. Go. Now. Kerstin makes it to the Delray Medical Center in about seven minutes, a little quicker than your average sirens-full-blast, skip-the-red-lights ambulance driver.

They rush you into the Emergency Room. The doctor on call orders a CT scan. The nurse draws blood through your new PICC line.

Doctors and nurses hover around you, waiting to solve a disaster that never comes.

Your lungs, liver, spleen, adrenal glands, and pancreas appear normal. Your gallbladder took a hike in 1981, and it has not returned. There's no bowel obstruction. The bladder remains partially distended (from the Great Catheter Wars). They cannot see the appendix clearly, but the lack of inflammation suggests no acute appendicitis.

"My appendix made it all the way to heaven in 1954," you tell them. "The plan I now have is to sneak past Saint Peter, one small piece at a time, organ by organ." The doctor smiles, but not much.

Everything on the CT scan appears relatively standard, even your kidneys. The new blood work flags no problems. The potassium level registers dangerously low in the old blood work, which set off all the alarms and sent us racing to the ER.

Potassium is an electrolyte, a mineral that occurs naturally in people. Fruits and vegetables are significant contributors. Bananas are famous for potassium. Hypokalemia (too little potassium) can bring your heart to your knees, stop it from contracting. You drop dead.

"We had to refrigerate the blood because the home care nurse forgot to take it with her," Kerstin tells the doctor. He rolls his eyes, shakes his head, walks off. Apparently day old, forgotten, refrigerated blood does not measure up to medical reality very well. You go home. The memory-challenged nurse who forgot to take the blood with her, for immediate analysis, never reappears.

Before leaving Florida Hospital Celebration, you both agree to continue using their doctors and offices during your recovery. You have no trust in your hometown primary doctors at Personal Physicians Associates. You have no confidence in Doctor Gottenger at Advanced Urology of South Florida. Right or wrong, you and Kerstin blame them, and their staffs, for kick-starting a medical journey you never planned and certainly never wanted.

Kerstin sends a six-page fax from the office to Doctor Shoaib Siddiqui the day after your false emergency. Five pages of medical stuff and the cover page below

Re: Temple Williams born 11/10/1942 Please find attached the Discharge Report for Temple Williams at the Emergency Room, Delray Medical Center in Delray Beach on Friday, August 3, 2012. The blood lab work and the report CT scan are also attached.

Temple and I will be driving up to Orlando on Monday, August 6, for a follow-up visit with Dr. Puskuri. We'll drive back to Boca Raton the same day.

On Wednesday, August 8th, Temple will drive up by himself for his appointment with you. I cannot accompany him due to a previous commitment. This worries me. He will be driving for over 6 hours that day. If there's any way you could see Temple (including any CT that needs to be done) on Tuesday, August 7th, the two of us could stay overnight at a hotel and relax together from Monday to Tuesday. If this is not possible, then we'll keep the appointments as they are.

On Monday, you and Kerstin head for Orlando. You have a Florida Hospital address, and you put it in the car's GPS. You hit a detour on the Florida Turnpike. Brush fires rage across central Florida. You smell them forty miles before you see them smoking in the distance.

You hit a detour on the detour.

Then you drive into a detour on the detour of the detour.

"Things are not going well," Kerstin says.

"Don't worry. It'll get worse," you reply. And, of course, it does.

You swing out to the west coast of Florida and then approach the Orlando area from there. After six hours, you finally roll into the address on the GPS.

You see no clinic, nothing that looks like a medical building. You phone. You have gone to an administrative office, although you do not see it anywhere.

But now rush hour has honked its way into Orlando. After seven and a half hours, you park in front of Doctor Puskuri's office in something that resembles a strip mall. It is not impressive.

As you enter the small reception area, you tell Kerstin that it has been a beautiful day for a drive in the country. Neither of you smiles. And Doctor Puskuri is not there.

"We've been driving almost eight hours," Kerstin says. The receptionist and a male nurse are polite, but they are not magicians. They cannot make Doctor Puskuri suddenly appear.

The male nurse has your medical information, and he starts to talk to you about kidney dialysis.

"What are you talking about?" you ask.

"You have renal failure," he answers, looking at the doctor's notes. "You're going to need to go on kidney dialysis."

"Like hell, I will," you say. It is the first time either one of you hears about kidney dialysis. Sure, the 13-day hospital stay at Florida Hospital beat up the kidneys a little, but dialysis? No way. The real problem is an infection. Fix the infection.

The male nurse seems a little confused, nervous that he has perhaps stepped over a medical boundary that he did not recognize. It is not the way a patient should find out he's stumbling into kidney dialysis.

Nobody at Florida Hospital Celebration even mentions it, although the fact that Doctor Puskuri was a Nephrologist, a kidney doctor, might have been a pretty good hint.

"Dialysis is not so bad," he tells you.

He tugs at his shirt, pulls the collar over his shoulder, shows you a lump somewhere near his collar bone.

It is the port through which they attach him to a kidney dialysis machine.

"I've been on it for a couple of years," he says. "I'm waiting for a transplant. Make sure you get on the transplant list right away."

"No way," you say.

They take a blood sample from you before you leave. Kerstin cancels the appointment with Doctor Siddiqui, and you drive back to Boca. It is a quiet, angry ride. You finally get home at ten in the evening.

"The trouble with kidney doctors," you tell Kerstin, "is that they just see and think of you like a kidney."

"It's the infection we have to beat," she says. "The Mersa."

"You bet," you say. "And once that's gone, my kidneys will fix themselves."

"You're going to be fine," she says.

Both of you retreat into the safety and the stupidity of denial.

"We need to put together a medical team here in Boca." Who wants to operate with doctors who live three or four hours away on a good driving day?

You target the Boca Raton Community Hospital, popular with many of your friends. It has an excellent reputation, and it's growing. It quickly becomes the Boca Raton Regional Hospital. You spend a lot of time analyzing your choices before making the decision, and you never regret picking what everyone now calls Boca Regional.

Kerstin sends Doctor Siddiqui a fax asking him to refer you to the offices of Doctor Donald Heiman and Doctor Marcelo Filizzola, specializing in infectious diseases, associated with Boca Regional. You have a good friend who has been fighting infection, successfully, for many years with these doctors. The friend and his wife have a wing of the Boca Raton Regional Hospital named after them, significant contributors to the hospital and beautiful friends.

They know good doctors when they see them. Doctor Siddiqui's referral is to Doctor Heiman, who has well over 30 years of experience fighting infectious diseases.

Doctor Puskuri agrees to refer you to Doctor Scott Cohen, a young Nephrologist attached to the Boca hospital who has published important research papers on diabetes and kidney problems. You spend a lot of time on the Internet and the phone with friends, narrowing your choices to these top physicians. They both have excellent reputations. They graduated from top-notch medical schools.

You keep your Primary doctor, and you keep Doctor Gottenger, although you will not use them for anything. You try to replace the Primary, but nobody wants the job. Everyone specializes in something and has no interest in just being a gatekeeper. One doctor who does consider it demands an up-front fee of several thousand dollars.

A meeting gets set up with Doctor Scott Cohen in his office. Kerstin is not there.

"I'm distraught that a male nurse in Orlando delivers the news that I am going to be on kidney dialysis," you tell him. You hope he will chuckle and say the male nurse made a stupid mistake. Doctor Cohen is a young, bright research doctor. You like him.

"You have renal failure," he tells you.

For a moment, you feel lost. It seems worse than the day Doctor Gottenger tells you that you have prostate cancer.

You do not know anybody on kidney dialysis, but you know what it is, and you know it's not fun.

You struggle to say something to Doctor Cohen, finally settling on: "And I have Mersa." Might as well get all the cards on the table.

"Yes, and Mersa."

"I do NOT want to go on kidney dialysis," you tell him. He sighs. He understands this. He takes his right hand and shrugs it in the air.

"Is the Vancomycin hurting my chances of avoiding kidney dialysis?" you ask. "Are the antibiotics killing my kidneys?"

He tightens his mouth. You used to know a boxer in the Marine Corps who did this just before he tried to deliver a knockout punch to an opponent. It was an obvious "tell," and you could lean back a little and then paste him to the canvas when his wild swing missed your chin.

"You are not going to avoid kidney dialysis," Doctor Cohen says.

Knockout punch. You are stunned. You are glad Kerstin is not here for this.

"Can we wait a while?" you ask. The doctor shrugs his shoulders, not with indifference, but with inevitability. You are a difficult patient, and you both know it. You go home and try to figure out some magical way you can solve this problem without dialysis. You spend a lot of time on the internet.

"I'm going to end up on kidney dialysis," you tell Kerstin. She says you will be fine. You spend two days not talking about it. Maybe it will go away.

Then you get another "emergency" call at home, this time from Doctor Scott Cohen himself. You have continued with home care and wonder who forgot to handle your blood correctly this time.

You drive down to the emergency room at the Boca Raton Regional Hospital but without the urgency of the earlier dash to the Delray Medical Center. It takes some time before the emergency physician on call, Doctor Terry Cohen, sees you. He is no relation to Doctor Scott Cohen.

"The home care nurse probably screwed up and didn't get my blood analyzed fast enough," you tell the emergency doctor. "The potassium levels are going to be a little wacky." A nurse appears and draws some blood. You wait in an examination room that the hospital refrigerates for any Eskimos visiting Florida.

Doctor Terry Cohen returns and says: "Potassium level is fine. You can go home." It is a moment of truth for you.

"You better check the creatinine level," you say without getting up. "I think maybe my doctor was worried about the creatinine level, too." He disappears back to his computer, and you can see him pick up the phone. You wait.

You have only just learned about creatinine levels. It's a measurable chemical waste molecule created by metabolism in muscles. The kidneys filter it out when you go to the bathroom.

Because muscle metabolism remains constant day to day, creatinine levels have become a good yardstick of how well your kidneys function. If the creatinine level goes up, your kidneys are impaired. The poisons in your body, generally eliminated through the kidneys, are not getting scrubbed out of your bloodstream. Keep it up, and you can poison yourself to death.

Sitting at his computer screen and talking to Doctor Scott Cohen on the phone, the emergency physician gets hold of the numbers. When you first saw Doctor Scott Cohen, a few days earlier, your creatinine level was 3.5. The normal range is between 0.6 and 1.3. The blood drawn by the home care nurse over the weekend shows 4.3. The current blood draw registers a creatinine level of 4.9, and Doctor Scott Cohen recommends admission for acute renal failure.

The emergency room physician calls Doctor Barish, the primary, for the go-ahead with the admission. They forward the phone call to Doctor Abreu, who tells him that someone else is on call for non-Humana patients. Not his problem. He hangs up the phone.

Doctor Scott Cohen appears in the emergency room. They need to admit you, and everyone seems to agree.

Doctor Cohen talks to another emergency doctor, and they recommend admission by the Hospitalist always on duty at the Boca Raton Regional Hospital.

Before that happens, the hospital makes another attempt to bring Doctor Barish's office on board, and Doctor Roy Cohen, the senior doctor at Personal Physicians Associates, agrees to the admission.

You get a red wristband that says you are allergic to Diclofenac.

They send you through the entry process and wheel you in a bed up to your room, which you share with a man named Fred. Kerstin has gone home to get your portable computer so you can work while in the hospital. You're still trying to get your latest real estate websites up and running.

You and Fred talk a lot. A curtain separates your hospital beds, and you have no idea what he looks like for the first three hours of your friendship.

"What are you in for?" you ask.

"Open wound in my back," a voice behind the curtain says. "The doctors can't get the damned thing to heal. What are you in for?". He sounds old, but chipper. You think you can joke around with him a little.

"Ten to twenty for manslaughter," you say. "But I swear to God she deserved it."

He laughs, then he hurts. "Please, don't do that," he says.

"Sorry." You exchange names and small talk, and after a while, he falls asleep. His doctors heavily sedate him.

Kerstin appears, and you whisper while Fred remains quiet behind the curtain. She leaves late in the afternoon. She'll be back in the morning. Some doctors come in and talk to Fred, and then go. One of the doctors comes back, then rushes out again. During the next five days, you learn that all of Fred's physicians rush in and out. They never seem to walk. They constantly hurry.

"They don't know what the hell they're doing," Fred complains after the doctor rushes back out on the day you meet. You still have not seen him. Some nurses come in and get him painfully (from the sounds you hear) out of his bed and into a wheelchair. They push him around the edge of the curtain.

He's a small man, pretty old, with sharp features. A dark hairpiece is slightly ajar on his head, and he reaches up and positions it perfectly with a quick flick of a finger.

He has done this often in his life.

"Fred," you say. "You're an extremely handsome man!"

He smiles and gives a little wave. "Damned right," he admits as they wheel him into the hallway. You spend five days together. You tell each other a lot of stories, many of them true. You laugh a lot.

"Don't do that."

"Sorry."

Those two statements punctuate your conversations throughout your shared days and into your nights. Fred lives in a big house in a subdivision filled with multi-million dollar mansions. He bought it because he wants the whole family to be together. You meet his daughter and grandchildren and various in-laws, and Fred is the patriarch, the leader of the clan. He is even older than you thought, in his early nineties. But Fred is tough, fighting for his life. You leave the hospital before he does. You hope he makes it back home to the family he loves.

Doctor Scott Cohen sees you every day. The head doctor from Personal Physicians Associates visits. You like Doctor Roy Cohen (no relation to Scott). He's tall, dynamic, deep-voiced with professional authority, someone you might easily trust.

Doctor Heiman, an expert on infectious diseases, visits. You have not yet made it to his office for your first appointment, interrupted by your emergency hospitalization. You like him.

The first day you are at the hospital, they give you a Rapid Test for MRSA, which shows negative. You do not need to transfer to an isolated room.

You and Fred remain roommates. The Vancomycin is beating back the MRSA. But you are anemic, you feel weak, and your kidneys are not doing their job.

The Boca Raton Regional Hospital becomes quicksand. The world of medicine begins to swallow your life.

You get a blood transfusion. It makes you feel much better. But just for a while.

Two days later, you get another blood transfusion. The positive effects do not last as long. "You have to go on kidney dialysis," Doctor Cohen tells you.

They will remove your beautiful new PICC line. It's a sound system for dripping Vancomycin into your heart, but the dialysis machine demands a river into your bloodstream, not a trickling creek.

The surgeon, Doctor W. Anthony Lee, who will install a much larger and more efficient port into your body, asks if you want a temporary one or a permanent one.

Silly question. "Temporary," you say.

"Temporary it is," he replies.

You will learn, quickly, the error of your ways. And ultimately, because every Warrior Patient needs a little luck, choosing a "temporary" fix turns out to be correct.

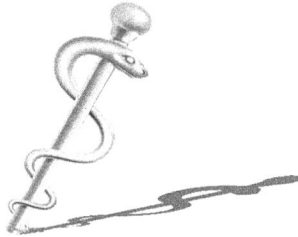

Warrior Patient Rule 9: Some physicians like to take a "mushroom" approach to their patients, believing that if they keep them in the dark, they will flourish. Smart patients live longer than dumb ones. _Good_ doctors appreciate this fact.

Chapter 10

Plug Into Dialysis

"I can't stand up," you gasp. Everything cramps. "I can't move."

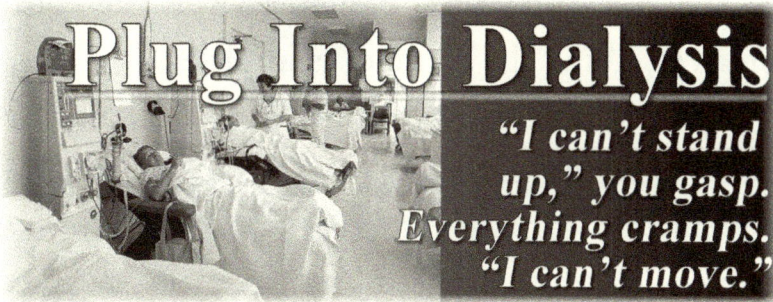

Doctor Rubio, the anesthesiologist, talks to you in the operating theater. You call him "my happy juice guy," and he puts up with your nonsense. "You should always be nice to anyone who can knock you out," he tells you.

You tell him you were a boxer in the Marine Corps, and you know exactly what he means. It comes out like this: *"I wath a botter inda Marny Kur an I canoe sackly whahoo mins."*

You are not entirely gone, but there is no pain, and the consciousness you feel is of floating, bright lights, cotton clouds, muffled noises. An X-Ray technician finds your jugular vein with a hand-held ultrasound. Then Doctor W. Anthony Lee, the surgeon, punctures the vein with a hollow needle. He runs a guidewire through the needle and into the vein, withdraws the needle, threads a catheter over the wire, removes it, and the catheter is in place.

It is much more complicated than this makes it sound. Doctor Lee is a skillful surgeon. He punches a beautiful hole in your chest, and after a lot of medical magic, you have a temporary port, a catheter ready, and waiting for a dialysis machine.

You come out of the fog, discover you are in a recovery area, drink orange juice, and get taken back to your room. You show Kerstin your port. Two small, flexible hoses come out of your chest, entry, and exit, closed with a single stitch, all protected by a flap of sterile white gauze.

"I can't swim with it, or take a shower with it," you tell Kerstin.

"No," she says. "But, you can certainly stay alive with it."

Over a century ago, in 1913, the world's first dialysis experiment was performed on a dog. In 1941, the world's first kidney dialysis machine for human beings included fifty feet of sausage skins, tin cans, odds and ends, and an old washing machine. Doctor Willem Kolff makes it in a remote Dutch hospital during World War II. The young inventor forges documents and scrounges materials under Nazi occupation to get his contraption built. Doctor Willem Kolff becomes the recognized Father of Dialysis.

By 1943, Doctor Kolff has a crude test machine completed. He treats over a dozen patients with acute kidney failure, and every one of them dies. The doctor keeps tinkering with it. In 1946, he operated on a 67-year-old-woman who was in a coma caused by acute renal failure. She regained consciousness. They say her first words were: "I want to divorce my husband."

She does, and she almost makes it to her 75th birthday before dying of something other than acute kidney disease.

By 1950, Doctor Kolff's invention has solved the disaster of acute renal failure. But very few doctors think it will work for patients with chronic kidney disease. They do not believe a human-made device can replace the extraordinary miracle of kidneys over the long term. The damage suffered by arteries and veins during the attachment procedure makes it extremely difficult to find new access points after just a couple of treatments.

Doctor Belding Scribner, a young professor at the University of Washington, solves the access problem when you are a Marine Corps recruit at Parris Island, North Carolina. He does it with a U-shaped shunt and plastic tubes, one to a vein, and one to an artery, using a new hi-tech material called Teflon®.

Doctor Scribner starts the world's first outpatient dialysis facility in January of 1962. The Seattle Artificial Kidney Center has six dialysis machines. Eventually, they rename it the Northwest Kidney Center.

Doctor Scribner paddles a red canoe from his houseboat to the center almost every day, and his vision establishes the outpatient model of dialysis that has become the standard of kidney care throughout the world. On June 19, 2003, he was presumed dead at the age of 82 when his red canoe was discovered, floating on the water in Seattle, empty.

There are over 5000 dialysis centers in America today. There's an average of about ten machines in each center, and there are also home dialysis machines. The Food and Drug Administration says that over 200,000 people actively use dialysis to treat their kidney disease.

At the Boca Raton Regional Hospital, they take your new entry port for a spin almost immediately. You later learn that this may be the only significant benefit of having a "temporary" rather than a "permanent" port into your bloodstream. Still in your bed, they wheel you into the corridor and over to the other side of the floor, to a room that contains two huge kidney dialysis machines.

They look a bit like mid-sized semi-computers from the turn of the century, filled with dials, screens, switches, buttons, and plastic spaghetti-like connection tubes. A large filtration canister well over a foot long snaps into the front of the machine. That's the artificial kidney, called a dialyzer.

You could probably cram over half a dozen real kidneys (they are about the size of an average fist) into one artificial one.

The dialyzer takes care of the blood filtering and waste removal that a healthy kidney does continuously (but it cannot produce hormones like a real kidney).

The dialyzer looks like a long plastic tube stuffed with elongated, ribbed vacuum cleaner filters inside of it.

Your blood passes through the filter membrane of the artificial kidney, which then catches a lot of the junk in your body.

Artificial kidneys are usually single-use items (although reusable ones do exist, especially for the home dialysis business).

They can cost up to $1,500 each.

Use them once, and then you toss them.

Kidney dialysis is a costly sport.

They have to give you a lot of proteins, an iron shot, and a thyroid-stimulating hormone because the artificial kidney can only clean up your blood. It can't do any of the miracle drug-making tricks of a healthy human kidney. You get another blood transfusion. You're good to go.

A technician covers you with warm blankets. You get cold when the blood passes through the machine and back into your system at the rate of about one cup a minute.

You shiver even though the humongous machine is programmed to keep your blood at the correct temperature. A nurse hooks you up. The plastic tubes start clear as they push blood-thinning medicine through the new doorway to your heart. The plastic tubing quickly turns red. Manufacturers program the machine to remove some fluid as well as waste material. There is no pain, no feeling of being emptied or sucked on. You fall sound asleep. After less than an hour, the giant machine starts beeping, waking you up. It is a piercing noise, a little frightening.

"Is the left engine on fire? Are we going to crash?" you ask the nurse.

She stares at you, puzzled, suddenly gets the airplane analogy, and laughs. "The engine is clogged," she says.

"You mean the dialyzer?" you ask.

Her eyebrows register surprise that you are on a first-name basis with some of the enormous kidney machine's moving parts. The artificial kidney has stopped filtering the waste that has been building up in you for weeks. The nurse pops open one of the connecting tubes, and it looks like thick, red glue. She clamps off the tubes attaching you to the machine. She yanks out the very expensive artificial kidney and smacks it a few times on the part of the device that does NOT say "Whack Here."

"I have an old power drill at home that also responds to that sort of treatment," you say, adding: "I guess there's so much junk in me I clogged the pipes?"

"Oh, no," she assures you, snapping the artificial kidney back in place. She throws away the tubing filled with your blood, which you think is a lot of piping and a lot of blood, and she starts over with new tubing. Juice it up. Turn it loose. The machine works for a few minutes and then suddenly starts beeping again. "I guess we need a new dialyzer," she says. "I'm afraid you're a clogger."

"But I'm still a pretty nice guy," you answer. She smiles, but she's not having fun. You are her last patient of the day.

You tell her that your original diagnosis up at the Florida Hospital near Orlando said you had a very high platelet count in your blood. Platelets are blood cells whose function is to stop the bleeding.

"So I clot easily," you say. "I think I'm about to become the Number One poster boy for dialyzer manufacturers."

The nurse shrugs with her mouth and then says: "It probably has more to do with the temporary catheter they put in your chest. They clog up a lot."

That's news to you.

The nurse plugs in a new artificial kidney, and you finish your first dialysis session smoothly. You don't feel any different when they wheel you back to your room across the hall, but you have shed a few pounds during the process.

"This is a great diet," you tell Kerstin. "You don't have to exercise at all. They just plug you in, and you lose weight."

"And stay alive," she adds.

"And stay alive," you repeat.

Doctor Scott Cohen stops by and tells you that everything went well. Then he says you will no longer be his patient.

Both Kerstin's and your voice answer in perfect unison: "Why?"

He laughs. "I'm moving to Washington, D.C.," he says. He has joined The George Washington Medical Faculty Associates. He wants to spend more time researching as well as practicing Nephrology.

He's probably in his mid-thirties, graduated from the University of Miami School of Medicine in 2001.

He will do very well, wherever he goes, whatever he does.

"Who's going to take care of me/him?" you ask, again in unison with Kerstin.

"Doctor Eric Lazar," he says. He's with the same medical group where Doctor Scott Cohen now works: South Florida Kidney Disease. You are about to meet the best doctor you ever knew, a model for the practice of medicine, and a man who might know how to build a road that can successfully lead a medical dope to healthy hope.

At your first meeting, you try to bite his head off.

You are angry. You feel trapped and cornered by kidney disease.

"Don't you dare tell me I can't get off dialysis," you say to him. You are in his examination room, and Kerstin tries her best to calm you down.

Doctor Lazar seems a bit shocked by this belligerent attitude.

His assistant, Ashley, inches herself closer to the doorway, an avenue of escape.

"I never said you would be on dialysis forever," he says. "Did I?"

"Don't you dare say transplant," you say, lowering your voice a little.

"There are many things we can do," he tells you. "But first, we need to eliminate a lot of the problems you have right now. You need to have kidney dialysis to get healthy enough to show us what can and cannot occur."

You calm down.

Doctor Lazar is a very tall, slender man, with sharp features and dark hair. Kerstin says he's good looking.

He graduates from and has qualification certificates from top medical schools. He moves smoothly for a man pushing 6'5".

His voice never rises above the level of logic and reason.

He might be able to build a road to recovery for you.

You think you should begin to trust him, but just a little.

Doctor Eric, as most of his patients call him, works with his father, Doctor Ira Lazar, who is also a Nephrologist and a very distinguished, silver-haired version of his son. There are several other doctors in their practice, and a Nurse Practitioner, who will play a role in your attempted recovery, Kathleen Custer. Call her Super Nurse. She has a master's degree (MBA) in nursing.

Their offices adjoin a dialysis center called Renal Associates of Boca Raton. They have a financial interest in it.

They have another office in Delray Beach, also attached to a dialysis center in which they have a financial interest.

"Not only is kidney dialysis an expensive sport," you tell Kerstin, "it also looks like a helluva profit center."

She says it's worth it, and you agree. You talk about a friend of yours who lives in a waterfront mansion in Fort Lauderdale, who owned a string of dialysis centers. He lives in "the house that kidneys built." He has a large, rectangular pool with a spectacular view of Florida's Intercoastal Waterway. It should have been a kidney-shaped pool.

There are 21 dialysis stations in the Boca Raton center where you receive treatment, and all of then circle a central command area.

A constant flow of nurses, patient care technicians, social workers, a dietitian, equipment technicians, and administrators move in and out of the command area.

Patients fill all 21 large dialysis chairs. Some walk, and some come in with wheelchairs, but most get into their dialysis stations on their own.

Some have to be winched in with a lifting mechanism.

In an entry area, patients ring a buzzer and wait. A technician lets them in when a station becomes available. A seemingly endless flow of customers fills all the stations.

The dialysis chair is comfortable, with a swing in TV set for entertainment. People bring their earplugs. People bring their blankets. People usually fall asleep during their three-to-five-hour kidney dialysis session.

You meet the leader of the central command station during your time slot, a nurse named Robin, who can juggle a dozen problems at once without dropping the ball.

She directs everything with an iron fist in a velvet glove.

Hardly anyone talks, unless it's to someone working at Renal Associates.

Friendships are rarely born in dialysis centers. A bond of silence casts its shadow over the dialysis stations: you are all in the same boat, and it is sinking. You cannot plug the holes, you don't know how to bail out the water, and you are heading towards a destination where none of you wants to go.

At Renal Associates, you are assigned the second chair beyond the door into the center. A commercial weight machine is on the wall across from the chair. You have a 6:45 AM slot time, three days a week. You watch people weigh in first, then move to their station. If they are in a wheelchair, they get pulled up on the commercial scales by a technician. The weight of their chair is measured and subtracted after they are safely at their dialysis station. Your weight becomes a critical yardstick in a dialysis center.

"Whoa, Jonathan," a technician says. "What were YOU eating and drinking over the weekend, buddy?"

"Nice job, Charlene, you haven't gained a single pound."

"Good job, Temple. You're now losing weight," a nurse tells you. "We're going to be able to figure out your dry weight pretty soon."

Dry weight is a critical yardstick. It's your weight without any excess fluid build up between dialysis treatments. It's the "ideal" weight a person would tip the scales at if they had a healthy kidney function.

The quest for dry weight is a painful one. On your first day at the dialysis center, you still weigh over 240 pounds. Your ankles swell (edema), and just about everything on you is stretched to record-shattering proportions (except Willie, who appears to have either hibernated or taken a long-term sabbatical).

At each session, you peel off more weight. A technician dials in a goal on the dialysis machine before you start and, while it's filtering out your poisons, it also takes away fluid. You weigh four or five pounds less after each session. The machines work in kilos because the best ones come from countries where the metric system dominates their numbers game. A kilo is 2.2 pounds. You're knocking off a few kilos during every session. You're keeping it off with proper dieting between sessions.

After each session, you have your blood pressure checked, standing up to make sure you can walk out of the dialysis center on your own. A few weeks into the program, a technician punches in the wrong numbers on your machine by mistake. Instead of stripping off one kilo, the dialysis machine takes off five. At the end of the session, the technician takes all your tubing and the throwaway artificial kidney and dumps it in a medical waste bin. Then he walks back to your station to help you to your feet and check your blood pressure. You bend into a ball.

"I can't stand up," you gasp. Everything cramps. "I can't move." You have had cramps in your life, but nothing comes close to this. Your toes curl. Your fingers curl. The pain is horrendous. The curling up of your body continues. Your legs cramp. Your thighs. Your arms. Your hair follicles. They are rushing to your station. They hang a saline solution on the pole and dump it into you through your catheter. A nurse is squeezing the bag to make it go faster. Then there's another bag. Your body begins to straighten out. You move to a wheelchair and roll to the side of the central command station. You get another bag of saline solution, and your legs and arms begin to relax. Slowly, your fingers and toes recover.

Robin is there. You talk about her husband cooking Caribbean "island food" for them that night. He's a great cook, she explains. Slowly, you make it back to your new normal.

"I think if I had a weak heart, I might have died," you tell Kerstin later.

Within a month, you hit your dry weight: 87 kilos, around 192 pounds. You pump your fist on the scale, get into your chair for the session. There's a commotion on the other side of the room. A patient erupts with the anger that remains just below the surface of many victims of kidney disease. Robin manages to quiet him down amid a flurry of extraordinary insults and foul language, which might have drawn you into the fray on her side a few years earlier. As she walks past your chair, silent tears reflect on her cheeks in the too-bright overhead lights.

"All we're doing is trying to help them," she tells a technician snapping in a new artificial kidney on your machine. "We're just trying to help them as much as possible. Why do they have to get so damned mad at us? Why mistreat us like this?"

The answer is in the questions: them and us. They are healthy, and you are not. A dialysis center is not a happy place. Nothing funny happens here. Laughter rarely invades the silence of serious illness — everything changes in your life. You often tell your friends it must be similar to being on death row. Only you get to go home at night. Physically, you feel like you've joined the walking dead after each session. Once you reach your ideal "dry weight," the deadening effect does not appear as often, but you have to remain at or near that weight.

Drink some soda pop or munch some crispy French fries between dialysis sessions.

Welcome back to the walking dead.

Things that used to be right for you, like wild rice, are suddenly wrong. White rice is acceptable. Eggs are right for you.

Fried calamari is out. How, you wonder, can anyone live without fried calamari?

You need a dietician to direct your table manners because the menu is no longer the one at your favorite restaurant.

Salt is a killer, and so is sugar.

Many dialysis patients have diabetes.

You can enjoy a cruise, provided it's on a dialysis boat. Such boats exist. They say they can be fun. Why not?

Everybody is in the same boat.

If you want to go on any trip, you must plan it months ahead of schedule. You must pre-arrange Dialysis centers wherever you go. Three times a week, for three to five hours. Have a lovely time. Send us a postcard of your dialysis machine. Wish you were here?

Don't think so.

Relationships change. One of your fellow kidney victims, a boisterous man, one of the few "talkers" in the room, speaks excitedly about his wonderful South American wife when you first meet him. The last time you see him, he tells you about their divorce.

Every time you go to the center for treatment, you look around the room and see the wreckage of kidney failure.

Getting a catheter in your chest turns out to be a mistake, although the "temporary" label associated with it seemed irresistible at the time.

A chest catheter can be used immediately after placement, but it requires longer treatment times at the dialysis center. It also has a higher infection rate, which can be fatal since the tip of the tube rests inside your heart. You can't shower with it, and it can destroy essential veins. It inspires clotting. You are King Clot, the poster boy for all of the dialyzer manufacturers in the entire world.

The best solution, called the gold standard of dialysis, is something called a fistula, which permanently connects an artery to a vein and installs beneath the skin, usually in a patient's arm. It provides better treatment, higher blood flow, fewer infections, fewer hospitalizations, and better survival rates (especially compared to catheters like yours). A fistula can last for 20 years. But the operation can take weeks or months to heal before a patient can use the fistula. You will eventually have this procedure if you cannot escape from dialysis.

"But I am going to make it out of here," you tell the nurses and technicians tending your machine. "Nobody escapes," some of them say to you. The rest of them turn away, avoiding the conversation altogether.

A few stations down from you, a doctor with kidney disease has a fistula. He bounces into the center with light steps and surprising vigor every day. His treatment lasts half as long as yours. He always quick-walks out of the center a few hours ahead of you. He is one of the few lively patients in the room. You decide you might be able to have a life with a fistula. He does.

A second choice is a graft, a tube that connects an artery to a vein. It's also permanent and beneath the skin, often used in patients with lousy veins. But it does not reduce the risk of infection or clotting, and it will not last as long as a fistula. Patients with a graft seem to have bruised and damaged arms.

The worst choice you can make is to have a catheter similar to the one in your chest. At the time, nobody explained this to you.

Perhaps they felt you needed to be on dialysis immediately, and the "temporary" solution became a necessity. You had renal failure, and you needed a quick fix into your heart. They pitched their offer so you would choose correctly.

You do not have to go to a dialysis center for treatment. You can do home dialysis. You and a family member (or caregiver) need some training to do it.

A neighbor chose this approach. He was tired of four-hour sessions three times a week at the dialysis center. His wife came home one afternoon. She heard the television going in the living room, figured he was getting ready for his dialysis session. His fistula disconnected. He was trying to do it himself, with no help. He bled to death.

Another method is called Peritoneal Dialysis (PD). It does not require a dialyzer. It uses a natural membrane in your body to filter waste from your blood. It requires a catheter that fills a natural cavity in your belly with a liquid that traps waste products and fluid. PD works round the clock. You just have to change your oil three or four times a day.

A fourth method is a kidney transplant. Over 26 million people in America suffer from chronic kidney disease. In late September 2014, over 123,000 people are on a list waiting for a kidney. In 2013, almost 17,000 transplants took place in the United States. Over 4,400 people die waiting every year in America. That's over 12 people a day.

Transplanted kidneys can come from family members, friends, or dead people who match your blood and tissue type. The waiting list for cadaver kidneys stretches out for years, and the kidneys do not last nearly as long as those from family or friends. Living kidney donors have very few complications, and the recovery only takes two or three weeks.

At least that's what they want the donor world to believe.

A very close friend of yours, Ric Nelson, tells you: "Temple, I will give you one of my kidneys for a transplant." It is a grand and sincere gesture of friendship.

"Do I have to promise not to beat you in tennis?" you ask.

We have a history of monumental matches, including one 76-game marathon that lasts over five hours. Ric goes in for triple bypass surgery a couple of days later.

"You're a tough friend," you tell him in the hospital, "virtually impossible to kill." He makes you leave because laughing hurts. His operation is a success, his recovery complete.

Ric's offer of a kidney is an extraordinary act of giving.

Our blood type matches, but you are not sure about the tissue type. Unfortunately, both his age (he's almost ten years older than you are and in fantastic shape) and his heart by-pass rule him out as a donor.

If you do get a kidney transplant, you will always need to take particular medicines to avoid rejection of the new organ.

Your life will change, almost as much as it does if you stay on dialysis. The most significant benefit is that a kidney dialysis machine is no longer tethered to your existence. You finally have a life.

A final choice is to stop treatment. You will die. A hospice can make the passage less painful, but you will die.

People with End-Stage Renal Disease (ESRD) are 13 times more likely to pull their plug than the general population. Not long after you start with kidney dialysis, this leads to an unusual conversation with a social worker at Renal Associates.

"How do you feel, Mr. Williams?" she asked, standing next to your dialysis machine with a notepad in one hand and a poised pen in the other.

"Please call me Temple," you say. "Mr. Williams was my father."

"Temple," she says with a pleasant smile. "How are you today?"

You smile back.

"Today," you say, "I am no longer afraid of dropping dead."

She sits down.

You can see all the alarm bells going off behind her eyes. You laugh. "Oh no," you say, "I'm not talking about suicide like my grandfather, who blew his brains out after my grandmother died."

You now have her undivided attention.

"Or my first cousin who shot himself in his sister's house." He was trying out for the Olympic ski team. He might have made it, but the team doctor ruled him out because he had a severe and fatal disease about which his mother had never told him. She knew, and he didn't. He killed himself.

The social worker is now sitting on the very edge of her chair.

"Or my mother, who took fifty sleeping pills ten years ago," you add.

"She woke up, and we saved her. Know what I told her? I suggested that the next time she wanted to do that, let me buy the pills. Get the job done right."

You belong to a tough, Irish family. Your mother thought this suggestion was pretty funny. You stayed with her 24-7 for many months until she ditched her suicidal tendencies.

She continued living a pretty good life, understanding that she was loved and needed by all her family.

On the other hand, the social worker looks like she's ready to call for help. Professional help.

Perhaps a beautiful, white straitjacket for the patient to whom she is talking.

"Listen," you say. "I have no thoughts of suicide whatsoever. I swear." She lowers her pad and pen, but it takes a while.

Her hands are showing early signs of essential tremors, a reasonably harmless disease your mother has passed along to her children. Or the social worker may just be nervous.

You smile at her. "I'm just not afraid of dying."

"Why not?" she asks.

"Because I've come close to death five times in my life, and I don't think it ever scared me. It was always more fascinating than frightening," you answer. "Except for the first time, which I don't remember too much about."

Warrior Patient Rule 10: When you sink into the quicksand of modern medicine, the only way out will be good doctors. Does this violate Rule 1? Not if you're up to your neck in medical quicksand. Grab the rope. Pull hard.

Chapter 11

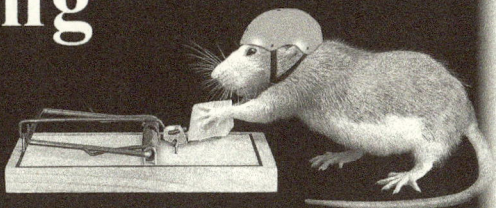

Cheating Death

She comes into your tent every day. She waits for the nurses to leave before she does this. That always takes time. When the women dressed in white appear outside of your tent, you roll over and stick your butt in the air. They put a needle in it. You never cry. It's part of the routine.

But your mother only comes into the oxygen tent when the nurses leave. She is not allowed to do this.

It does not stop her.

Her face is always wet with tears. You are dying, and this is your first memory of living. You do not remember coughing or feeling bad or having a fever or deadly pneumonia, but all of that is there. In 1946, pneumonia remained a death sentence for small children. You are not quite four years old.

Eighteen years earlier, Sir Alexander Fleming isolates a mold that can destroy a severe bacterium. Doctor Fleming names the mold penicillin. It is not until 1939 that Dr. Howard Florey, a future Nobel Laureate and three colleagues at Oxford University, conducts research that demonstrates penicillin's ability to kill infectious bacteria. On July 6, 1941, Doctor Florey and a fellow scientist from Oxford, Doctor Norman Heatley, arrive in America with a small amount of penicillin.

In the end, it is a rotten cantaloupe from a Peoria, Illinois fruit market that produces enough penicillin to start clinical trials in 1943. Penicillin production scales up for Allied soldiers wounded on D-Day. As they make more of it, the cost drops from priceless in 1940, to $20 a dose in 1943. It plummets to about a half a dollar a shot when you lift your butt to the women wearing white costumes in 1946. You are among the first children saved by penicillin, but all you remember is your mother sneaking into your oxygen tent in the hospital, and feeling her warm, wet cheek on your face. You do not die, thanks to good doctors, sound research, and functional medicine.

Your next two brushes with death occur because of raging hormones. The first time, you and your older brother are having a contest to see who can make love to a girl first. Philip has just turned sixteen, and you are a year and a few months younger. He has a driver's license, and it gives him greater mobility and a place in which to operate.

You are devastated the evening he pulls up in your father's red Willys Jeep station wagon, steps out of the driver's side and announces that he has "done the dirty deed." He is swinging a used prophylactic with his hand like a propeller, smiling. Your father steps out of the house, and Philip lets the proof of his accomplishment go. It flies up, streaking high in the bright glow of the porch light. It arches perfectly into the branches of the elm tree in the middle of the circle drive.

"Temple," your father says, staring at the swinging prophylactic twenty feet off the ground, "get in the house." You are too young for this sort of stuff.

If they only knew what they didn't know.

It is clear to you that successful sex requires car keys. A few nights later, you steal your father's Oldsmobile. You have an exciting and strenuous rendezvous with your first love on a blanket behind her father's tool shed, ten miles from your house along country roads. You are both fourteen years old, but you are closer to fifteen than she is. You are lovers for several years. Your friendship lasts much longer. As you grow older, you joke that both of you are guilty of statutory rape. Your statute of limitations in Ohio expires almost 40 years ago. The last time you see her is in the mid-1980s when she visits Kerstin and you in your loft in not-yet-trendy Soho, Manhattan. Afterward, you walk her to a cab on Greene Street and Houston, a half a block from where you and Kerstin live. She tells you that Kerstin is spectacular, but you already know that.

"I'm thinking of marrying my second husband again," she says. Her first husband is a drug addict, and she wakes up next to his dead body one morning and has a tough time getting over it.

Her second husband is a good man. They separated for a year, then divorced.

"I think that would be great," you tell her. You don't expect ever to see her again. They do re-marry, and then she divorces a second time. She meets many good men in her life, surrounded by children and grandchildren and a family who love her dearly. Many years later, you become Facebook and Twitter friends, and you share a lot of laughs.

On that long-ago first night, you get in your father's Oldsmobile and race home to tell your brother you are following in his glorious footsteps. You are finally a man, a fourteen-and-a-three-quarter-year-old man.

You are going 110 miles an hour when the car careens off the road. It tears through over two hundred yards of wooden fence posts and uproots four pine trees.

You flip the car over three times and end up in the back seat, tasting the metal from the fillings in your teeth.

You remember climbing into the back seat as soon as the long wooden fence posts start popping over the hood. You watch, fascinated, as the accident unfolds. The engine ends up in the front seat, where you had been driving. An electrical wire burns a small line into the left side of your face, but you do not remember receiving an electrical jolt. It is your only injury. The car is totaled. You walk over six miles along County Line Road, back to a homecoming that is not much fun.

Two years later, your raging hormones send you plummeting into a gorge 12 miles outside of Hot Springs, Virginia. Your grandfather has a farm there, with cows and sheep and pigs and plow horses, a magical place nestled in the Blue Ridge mountains. You are sixteen, going on seventeen, and you are much more interested in the nightlife at The Homestead, a famous resort in Hot Springs than you are in being on the farm. Everyone at The

Homestead is on vacation, having a good time. There is one young woman, a college freshman two years older than you, who feels she has to teach you things that only older women can teach a young man. You are an enthusiastic student, and after almost 24 hours of partying, you finally fall asleep when you are three miles from the farm. You are driving back home alone, along a dirt road that follows the Jackson River through a treacherous gorge. It is a slow-motion slide off the side of the mountain. You have a sudden and rude awakening; then, everything moves faster as your father's brand new station wagon careens through the tops of trees towards the Jackson River 50 feet below. This time you are hurt. You walk the three miles back to the farm after climbing out of the gorge. You stumble into your parents' room at 6:30 in the morning, and your mother screams when she sees you covered in blood. Your father says: "Shut up, Lyd! He'll be fine!" You drop to the floor. Everything after that comes in broken film clips of memory. Hospital lights. A train station platform. An overnight sleeper back to Ohio. At home downstairs with your father in an enclosed porch that you call The Green Room.

"You're going to pay for the car," your father tells you.

No argument. You work construction, give three-quarters of what you earn to your dad for two summers. You work overtime. You pay everything off. He also collects insurance on the total wreck. Your father, a partner and senior bond salesman, is occasionally a smart guy.

You never have another car accident. Never come close. Neither of your brushes with death behind the wheel scares you. They only fascinate you. Perhaps time smoothes their sharp edges.

In 1964, you became a subway cop in New York City. You do it as an investigative reporter for an afternoon newspaper called *The New York World-Telegram & Sun.* The police department never knows you are a reporter until after you turn in your gun and your badge. The newspaper returns the money you earn as a cop to New York City. Your bylined seven-day, front-page story titled "I Was a Subway Cop" shows what it is like to wear the blue uniform of a policeman in America's largest metropolis. You write about the Police Academy.

You tell the story of trying to save the life of a civilian in Grand Central Station. You make your first arrest.

As the story runs, you live under an assumed name in lower Manhattan (the idea of

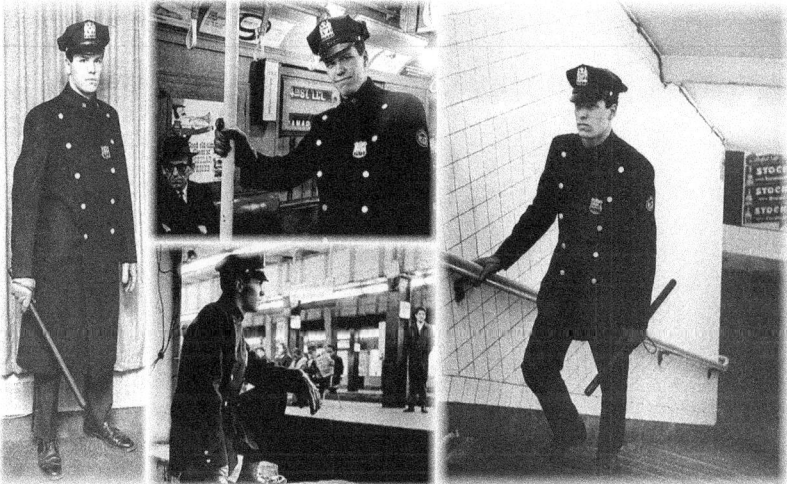

Photos by Stanley Wolfson, staff photographer, *New York World Telegram and Sun*, 1965, 7-day series: "I Was A Subway Cop" by Temple Williams

your editor, Richard Peters). You meet with the District Attorney of New York City. Some of your fellow cops lose their jobs because of what you reveal. Some face prison.

You cannot go near your apartment on East 4th Street because you are a target, considered a traitor by many of the cops.

They break into your ground-floor apartment and hang your two pet cats from a light fixture in the ceiling.

You leave the city, traveling to New Orleans to stay with your oldest brother, Scott.

You get a phone call there early one morning.

"It's for you," Scott says, handing you the phone. Muffled voices make meowing sounds, followed by group laughter, followed by a dial tone. There is no call identity in those days, but it does not take a scholar to figure out what is going on.

You return to New York City a month later. Phone calls threaten your life. On your way to work at the newspaper one morning, a policeman in the subway draws his gun and holds it down to his side, almost invisible to people on the subway platform. He asks you why you did it.

"Why I did what?"

"Why did you stab my friends in the back?" he says. He is smiling, but it is not a friendly smile. He is angry.

"I didn't do that," you say. "The bad cops all stabbed themselves."

A subway roars into the station. The cop raises his gun slightly, but not pointing it at you, although you remember his hand is shaking. You keep looking at his weapon, not at him. Some people get off the train and quickly moved aside. You step back into the subway car, watching the gun, careful not to trip.

The doors close. The cop never stops smiling, but the train moves. You think this policeman is probably someone who hangs skinned cats from ceilings, and you can feel your heart beating. You taste metal in your mouth. But you don't think you are ever scared. Just fascinated, waiting for him to raise the gun, waiting for an explosion that never comes.

At least that's what you tell yourself, often, until you finally believe it.

"Did you know him," your editor Richard Peters asks.

"I don't think so," you say. "Maybe the guy was in my class at the Academy."

"What was his badge number?" he asks.

"Smith and Wesson," you reply to Richard Peters. "38-caliber." That's what you all pack back in those days.

"Get his name, Williams."

You never try.

You remember going down a floor from the City Room that day, walking past the clickety-clack of all the typesetters and their huge machines (digital has not yet turned print journalism into a computer game). You walk into a small, windowless area that you called the Skeleton Closet, the obit room.

You smile at the woman in charge and ask her if you can read your obituary. "Who are you?" she asks.

"Temple Williams," you say.

"Oh ... the cop."

"The ex-cop," you say. The woman doesn't seem to like you. Maybe she is married to a cop or has friends on the force. She inks up your obit, presses it onto some paper, and hands it over. They have it there, ready to go in case something happens to you. It is a pretty ordinary obit, using a small photo of you as a cop with the hat knocked back on your head a little. Nice touch. You wonder who wrote it.

"It doesn't say how I died," you say. The woman smiles, but she does not laugh.

You receive two nominations for the Pulitzer Prize, once for the seven-day series, and once for an article in the series, called: "To Save An Old Man." Which you try to do in Grand Central Station because you're a good cop, and the other two cops who are with you will not give a collapsed old man mouth-to-mouth resuscitation. "He doesn't even have a pulse, kid," one of the cops tells you. But when the emergency crew arrives, he does have a pulse. You bring him back. After the story runs, his family calls you up at the newspaper and says thanks to you. He died in the hospital after you saved him.

The World-Telegram & Sun started its death throes as a newspaper in 1966. A prolonged newspaper strike helps push it over the edge. You have a vague opportunity to work for the International Herald Tribune, or you can take a small pile of money and get out of town.

You take the money. You go and live in Africa for six years, where you see death for the fifth time in your life. It hangs around you for three or four weeks. You spend time in East, Central, and Southern Africa, seeing things you have never seen before, smelling things you have never felt before. You love Africa. It has its own, pungent odor, its unique sounds, its strange forms of life, and death.

You are on Hell's Run, a long, mostly dirt road which runs from Dar es Salaam (Bay of Peace), once the capital of Tanzania, into Lusaka, still the capital of Zambia. You are under a tarp that holds down a massive bladder of gasoline on the back of a tanker truck. The smell of petrol is strong, but your speed along the rough, dirt road keeps you ventilated.

You are approaching a border checkpoint near the Great Rift Valley, where you will cross into Zambia.

The driver of the tanker truck is helping you get out of Tanzania, where your visa has expired, and people who are not your friends want to prove that they are not your friends. You are not sure he has received enough money to keep his mouth shut at the border crossing. You're feeling a little light-headed from the petrol fumes.

"*Nice siku kwa ajili ya kuendesha, rafiki yangu,*" the border guard says. Swahili. Nice day for a drive, old friend.

"Ndiyo," says the driver. "Na hakuna mtu alijaribu pigo me up."

They laugh loudly. Nobody tries to blow his truck up today.

A lot of tanker trucks explode in a ball of fire on Hell's Run, but it's usually because the drivers fall asleep, not because of sabotage or tracer rounds. The drivers get paid by the trip, not by the hour. It's good money in a nation where jobs are tough to find. Some of them drive 48 hours without a break. Burned-out hulks get pushed off the side of the road, torched skeletons along the Bukhoro Flats bordering the mountains in the Mbeya region of Tanzania. The gasoline must get through to Lusaka. Prime Minister Ian Smith has closed the border to Rhodesia (now Zimbabwe). Zambia is starving for energy. Gas goes into Lusaka in huge tarp-covered rubber bladders, and copper comes out as payment.

On the truck in which you are hiding, gears suddenly shift. You move past the border post. Another similar stop in Zambia, only they speak English. The same laughter, the same patter, and then you are through. You get off the truck another five miles down the road.

"Asante kwa ajili ya kuokoa maisha yangu, bwana mkubwa," you say to the driver. Thanks for saving my life, great master. "Bwana mkubwa" is a little over the top, but he likes it and laughs, cranking the truck back into gear, disappearing in the dust towards Lusaka.

You walk into Malawi. You have some friends in Blantyre, the capital, and there is no border crossing. It takes you a week to get to Blantyre, where the police arrest you before you can find your friends. You have malaria, and you have a touch of dysentery. The only thing you don't have is a visa.

You spend a day being interrogated by the secret police, one man, in particular, who keeps asking you if you know about the horrors of Zomba Prison.

You keep asking him about the joys of being taken to the American Embassy. Nobody laughs. They will not let you go there.

They accuse you of being a spy and put you on a plane to Salisbury, Rhodesia. They do not know you have come from Tanzania.

You have carefully removed the page with Tanzania's expired visa from your passport, even though the pages have numbers.

In Rhodesia, the Criminal Investigation Department (CID) arrests you at the airport and holds you overnight. They accuse you of teaching people in the Mozambique Liberation Front (FRELIMO) how to blow things up.

"Why would I do that?" you ask the CID interrogator staring at you.

"Because it is something the United States Marine Corps has taught you to do, Williams," he replies.

Now, how the hell do they know that?

The Rhodesian Police drive you up to portable stairs leading to an old DC-3 airplane the following morning. "Where am I going?" you ask them.

"Back to Malawi," they say.

And now you know you are going to die. Nobody comes out of Zomba Prison, not back in those days. The only way you leave is in a pine box or through the back door to feed the crocodiles that wait for the dead.

The plane lands at Chileka Airport, which is nine miles outside of Blantyre. You are the last person to get off. There is nowhere to hide on a DC-3. The man in the secret police who spends so much time interrogating you earlier is standing at the gate, smiling at you.

You walk up to him, hold out your hand, and say: "I never really caught your name."

"My name cannot be caught," he says with great seriousness. You have no idea what he means, but it does not sound very friendly. He does not shake your hand. He does agree, however, to take you to the American Embassy before going to Zomba Prison.

A few years ago, you wrote an article in a book commemorating (posthumously) the one-hundredth birthday of your Godfather, Kenyon C. Bolton, II. It's an excellent way to explain what happened in Blantyre, Malawi, and how and why you survived the ordeal because of something called "A Kenny Moment."

It was, and remains, a glorious club - being a Godchild of Kenny Bolton. Uncle Ken scattered grand moments into every corner of the mind, every facet of life.

My father's best friend became one of my best friends and the Best Man at my first wedding. It took three of my largest Ushers, and a good deal of discussion, to remove him from the wedding car as the reception faded into dusk. He insisted that he was part of the honeymoon.

Ken was always magic for me. He was an adventure, Africa, France, unknown things that combined whispers with laughter, turning random moments into unforgettable memories.

Uncle Ken inspired love and joy whenever we met. My bride of almost 40 years, Kerstin, was hopelessly enraptured by him after about 30 seconds of their first meeting. So much so that we now have "Kenny Moments" in our lives.

That's what we call them. Often in unison.

A "Kenny Moment" can contain anything from caviar and champagne to the spectacular stillness of a Florida sunset in the Keys.

It can be walking in a land you've never seen before and never thought you would. Kenny Moments are what make life fun, different, exciting.

Sometimes they can change your life.

It was my second year in Africa and my twenty-fourth on earth. As an ex-Marine and an ex-NYC cop, I was invincible. I was also on my way to the Zomba High-Security prison in Malawi, as an inmate, not a visitor.

I had managed to get a message through to my father via the bored and mostly indifferent American Embassy in Blantyre, the capital of Malawi. His youngest son was in trouble.

People did not survive well in the Zomba High-Security Prison.

My father contacted his best friend, my Godfather Uncle Ken. He contacted his mother, Frances Payne Bolton. She had become a Congresswoman in 1939 when she served out the last year of her deceased husband, Chester's term.

Frances Bolton won the congressional seat in Cleveland's 22nd District on her own in 1940, the first woman from Ohio to do so. She served in Congress for almost three decades (29 years to be exact). She focused on nursing and foreign affairs.

She was the principal reason this nation graduated 125,000 Cadet Corps nurses during World War II (thanks in large part to the Bolton Act). In 1945, 85 percent of the nurses in America were Cadets, equal in status, and pay to a full-commissioned military officer.

In 1966, Congresswoman Francis Payne Bolton (as head of African Affairs) contacted the bored and indifferent American Embassy in Blantyre, Malawi.

Miraculously, Uncle Kenny's wayward Godson went from being Zomba Prison inmate into an honored guest of the Government of Malawi.

Sometimes, "Kenny Moments" save your life.

When I was very young, my Grandfather on my mother's side told me that if I walked into the woods and sat down and did not move a muscle for 30 minutes, I might see something I had never seen before. I figured he was just trying to shut me up. But now, decades later, I realize he was defining, almost correctly, a "Kenny Moment."

My dear Godfather, Uncle Ken, gave me the greatest gift of all. He gave me the Joy of Life and taught me that it had no strict definitions, no hard and fast rules. It has love, and laughter, and joy, irregular sharp edges, and always a lot of surprises.

Every life should contain many "Kenny Moments."

And so you survive your fifth brush with death, and you say you have no fear of it (although bravery is always easy when you are still on the right side of the grass).

You prefer to treat death as an old acquaintance, a thread of continuity entangled in the net that stretches across your life.

Your journey from medical dope to healthy hope still has a long way to go. But you are willing to smile at death, ready to tell it an old joke: You have nothing against funerals, you just don't want to go to your own.

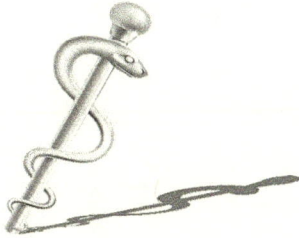

<u>Warrior Patient Rule 11:</u> Death makes people edgy, and healthy folks do not like ill people. So plan your "sick" conversations very carefully. And make sure there's a "for better or worse" clause in your marriage vows.

Chapter 12

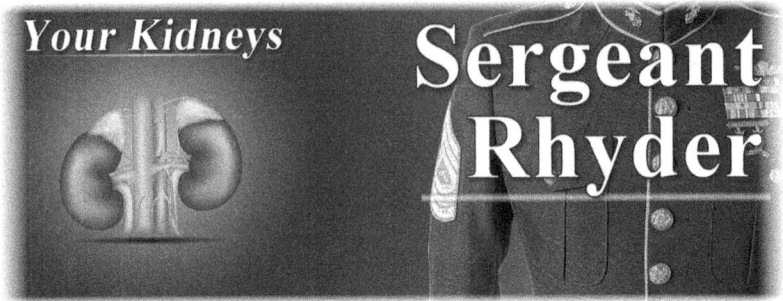

Your Kidneys — **Sergeant Rhyder**

This chapter is about your kidneys, but it starts with Staff Sergeant Rhyder, your Marine Corps Drill Instructor at Parris Island in 1961. He is one of the fiercest warriors you will ever know. On parade day, Korea splashes across his chest. Purple Heart. Silver Star. Battle commendations and campaigns. It is before Vietnam, before Granada, before Iraq, before Afghanistan.

Sgt. Rhyder teaches you how to fight. He decides to volunteer you as his representative in the company boxing championships.

He moves you up from middleweight to heavyweight, and you do OK. You have the moves. You can dance in the ring. You have some fear, but it is a reasonable fear, caution that you can quickly turn into aggression. Your last memory as a Marine Corps boxer is this thought: "Don't drop your head into a southpaw's uppercut." You have never been hit so hard in your life.

You wake up in the infirmary. Sgt. Rhyder is scowling at Parade Rest at the foot of your bunk. "You did OK, kid, made it through three rounds. You were boxing a semi-pro out of Philadelphia. I never thought you'd make it through one round. You did OK."

It is the kindest thing that Sgt. Rhyder ever says to you.

Sgt. Rhyder believes in toughness and discipline and cross-training before it is ever called cross-training. He wakes you up at 2 am and marches you with full gear through the swamps and wastelands of South Carolina. He double times you five miles before you can make your morning call in the latrine. He slams you through an obstacle course for an hour and a half in the scorching midday Carolina sun. Different times of day and night. Different challenges. Your metabolism changes. Your body hardens.

Cross-training makes good Marines.

Fast forward to your kidney failure. You have been on dialysis for well over three months now, with a man who you think might be one of the best kidney doctors in the world.

Exceptional nurses and dialysis technicians care for you.

The odds of kidney recovery remain a long shot, and some say as much as 1000 to 1. But the more likely number is 100 to 1. There are no guidelines for what they call renal recovery (RR), only the fact that it is scarce.

End-stage renal disease (ESRD) is total and permanent kidney failure. Between 1980 and 2009 (the latest statistics you have), it jumps nearly 600 percent. In the United States, 871,000 people suffer from this debilitating disease.

At the end of 2009, patients on dialysis number 398,861, and an additional 172,553 have a working, transplanted kidney.

Over 100,000 new patients join their ranks every year.

The number of renal failure deaths rises from 10,478 in 1980 to 90,118 in 2009. Treating end-stage renal disease patients costs the United States over $40 billion in public and private funds in 2009.

Recovery of your damaged kidneys is so rare that very few medical experts bother with clinical studies. There's a Swedish one that analyzes a single person. An Australian study takes a look at eight renal recovery patients.

From the beginning, you have fought for your kidneys. A surprising number of dialysis patients limit their physical activity to watching television, reading books, talking to friends and family, anything other than physical exertion.

When you can barely walk, you walk. You often do it late at night under the street lamps in your community, when nobody else is around. You are embarrassed to show your neighbors how feeble you have become. You carry two small, powerful flashlights. Stopping at the crosswalks feels especially dangerous. You lose your balance when you have to stop. You walk with your legs wide apart, making it less likely that you will fall over. Sgt. Rhyder remains a ghost in the background. The guardian warrior never smiles. If the edges of his mouth twitch up a bit, it almost always heralds an unpleasant moment. There are many.

At first, after each dialysis treatment, you return home and collapse into bed, unable to move. You remember when the technician dials in the wrong numbers that send you into cramps, head to toe. The event is an epiphany. You choose to either accept what many consider to be the death-row life of a dialysis patient or get up off the canvas and fight. Not with words or thoughts.

Brains are not enough.

Sgt. Rhyder is at the foot of the bed, standing at parade rest, watching.

One day you when you come into the dialysis center, a patient called "Judge" is being wheeled out on a gurney by the Emergency Services people. You like the Judge. His body is crippled into a wheelchair, but he is tough (yes, he had been a judge). He is very old, but an angry fighter.

They take him to the hospital. He returns a few days later. As they wheel him back into the dialysis center, you start to applaud his arrival. Others join in.

It is the only time you ever see the Judge twinkle a bit, a spirited smile curling his lips, lifting his head ever so slightly from its hangdog position. His left hand lifts a few inches off his wheelchair's armrest, tries to wave, makes it. The entire room hears the applause, lifting its collective spirit briefly higher.

Two days later, the Judge checks into a hospice, takes himself off dialysis, has morphine dripped into his veins. He dies. He has fought a good fight, but he has become worn out.

You know that you have to escape the stranglehold of dialysis, and you know it will hurt. It will take Marine Corps stuff.

You start to bike to the dialysis center - a six-mile round trip—three times a week. None of the staff ever remembers anyone doing such a foolish thing. Biking home after the treatment is like stumbling through a marathon with crazy glue on the bottom of your running shoes.

The first day you peddle to the dialysis center, CeCe opens the door when you buzz to enter. She is one of the nurse technicians who help you in and out of your assigned chair. She is tall, regal, both in stature and looks. Shadows of an ancient Ethiopian princess emanate from her. She stares at your bike helmet and your rain gear covered with reflective tape.

"What are you doing, Mr. Williams?"

You are a little out of breath and unsteady. "Biking," you say.

"You can't do that," she says.

"I just did. I'm here."

You unload your backpack, which holds a 17" portable Vaio computer and a heavy blue blanket to keep you warm in the chair.

"Who's going to pick you up and take you home?" CeCe asks.

"My bike," you say.

She shakes her head at such foolishness. You have lost your mind.

After three and a half hours of dialysis, you stand up, not feeling very stable. You get your blood pressure taken, stuff the computer and blanket in the backpack, and get suited up for the ride home. You struggle to the elevators that will take you to the ground floor.

You half walk and half stumble across the covered entryway to the tree where you have locked your mountain bike. You stand there, balancing unsteadily on wide-apart legs, looking at it for a long time.

You did not know a mountain bike could scare you.

You unlock it from the tree, put on your helmet. You will take sidewalks all the way home. You will not risk going out on the road, which you did when you biked to the center.

You almost fall over, getting on the bike.

You do not remember riding home.

But one of your good friends does.

"I saw you, on the sidewalk, inside the subdivision," Alan Klein says. "You were on your bike, not moving, and you had your arms around a tree, hanging on to it with one hand and your other hand was on the handlebars of your bike."

Alan is worried.

You seem frozen to the tree in the morning heat of Florida.

He walks up to you and asks: "What are you doing?"

"Biking home," you say.

"Do you want me to help you?"

"Biking home," you repeat, tightening your grip on the tree. Perhaps you can take the tree with you.

"I can help you home," Alan says. He worries about your sanity and your safety.

"I'm fine as long as I'm on the bike," you tell him. "I can balance on the bike. It's the stopping and starting that's hard. And getting off the bike."

You let go of the tree, almost fall, start pedaling, catch your balance with some help from Alan, and head for home a quarter of a mile away.

You do not remember how you get off the bike, but you make it, go indoors, collapse on the bed, and quickly fall asleep.

It is your very shaky start to what eventually will become a 20-mile bike ride every day. After a month, you are pedaling almost 200 miles a week.

"So your numbers are coming down," Doctor Eric Lazar says. The tall, elegant man, deliberate in every way, explains everything, often with words containing far too many syllables. He always does it with care and often with hope. "The numbers are creeping lower, and that is a positive sign."

The Dietician, Michele Geraci, wheels her chair over to your dialysis station.

"I forgot to get you the gold stars," she says. "Do you want me to get the gold stars?" You smile your best 70-year old smile and tell her not to worry.

The dietician's news is all good. The strange diet is working. Lots of protein, lots of eggs, no salt. No orange juice. No bananas. Strawberries and blueberries are OK. Starfruit will kill you. It will. It will end your life.

You have gold stars in every dietary category. You feel pretty good. You decide that you will follow Michele and her strange advice through the gates of hell.

"Your creatinine level keeps creeping lower, and that's a good thing," Doctor Lazar repeats a week later. It has been up to 5.5 - renal failure - and has dropped to 3.7 over two months. Then 2.9. Then 3.1. Then 2.9 three weeks in a row.

"We're going to give you a 24-hour urine test," Robin tells you in the dialysis center. "You save it in this orange jug for 24 hours, and then they analyze it to see what, if any, toxins are taken away by your damaged kidneys."

You considered asking close friends and family pets to join you in this endeavor, but figure it might not be a joke.

Most dialysis patients don't pee. Their fist-sized kidneys just stop functioning. You have two kidneys, one on either side of your spine at the bottom of your rib cage. Each one contains close to a million filtering units called nephrons. Each nephron contains tiny blood vessels. Each nephron acts like a miniature blood-cleaning factory attached to a small hollow tube. Blood passes through the factory, gets cleaned, and chemicals and water get added or removed in the hollow tube according to your body's needs. The end product of this miraculous assembly unit gets eliminated from your body as urine. And you have almost a million of them chugging away in each kidney, a MILLION cleaning factories. It boggles the mind.

When your kidneys fail, dialysis takes over the filtering but not the "chemicals" job of the tiny nephrons (that requires separate medicine from your doctor, hormones, and iron and things like that).

Without dialysis machines, people with failed kidneys poison their bodies quickly and die an unpleasant death.

That's what the Judge did when he took himself off dialysis.

He understood this. The morphine drip helped ease his passage.

You consider him a brave warrior.

You return the big orange jug to Robin. The 24-hour urine analysis shows that your kidneys are functioning in a limited way. Not great. But your tiny nephron factories have not all gone on strike.

"So now we're going to see what happens when you skip a dialysis session," Doctor Lazar tells you several weeks later. Holy smokes!

"You're going to take away my big, mechanical, whirling security blanket and hope for the best?" you ask the Doctor.

"You can always go back on the machine in an emergency," he says.

It is what you are working for, biking for, walking for, doing pushups for, and taking steroids for. Now it's here. It seems too sudden.

They will closely monitor everything. Later that night, you watch an ad on TV from a class action lawyer who wants the survivors of dead dialysis patients to join in a suit against sudden death due to dialysis. You do not write down the phone number.

You have reached your ideal "dry weight," and you are maintaining it.

You no longer look like a walk-on for the Macy's Thanksgiving Day Parade. You have lost almost 70 pounds. You are back to your decades-old Marine Corps fighting weight. The battle is on. You can practically smell the grease in the air, hear the bee-sting snap of live ammunition passing overhead.

"Make sure you keep taking the prednisone," they say. It's a popular steroid, usually administered at less than 5mg a day. You are taking 60mg every morning. It makes your face a little rounder, you might gain some weight, and you have dreams where you meet a lot of the dead people you have known in your life.

You have one dream that repeats itself. You are in a field in Mozambique surrounded by scrub brush. A Portuguese soldier that you did not kill, although you could have, walks up to you and wants to show you a picture he has in his hand. You think it is going to be him, shot, or his family dead, but it is not. It shows him with a dog, sitting in front of a small white farmhouse and they are smiling, even the dog smiles with its tongue hanging out. It is a very goofy-looking dog, but huge. The photograph is also large, not just a snapshot, and it is spotless. You don't want to touch it because you are very dirty, as is the Portuguese soldier. You wonder how he keeps the photograph so clean. He does not leave any smudge marks on it. You and the soldier talk. He chatters away in Portuguese, and you understand everything he is saying, although you only know a handful of words in that language. You speak to him in English and broken Swahili, which you know he doesn't talk, and he understands you perfectly. When you wake up, you cannot remember what you are talking about, only that it is crucial. You have variations of this dream four times, and you think you have the same conversation each time. After the first dream, you know it is essential to try to remember the conversation, but you never manage to remember what you discuss.

It is a surprisingly comfortable dream.

Your kidneys like prednisone, it reduces inflammation, and that helps them function better. You don't take it forever. It's just a kick start, part of the road to recovery that Doctor Lazar has carefully built.

So you skip a treatment, and you walk, you bike, and you lift light weights. You pray a lot, and so do many of your friends.

And God says: "Yes."

The creatinine level holds at 2.9. Other levels improve slightly.

You do not gain any weight.

"So now you're going to come in and have another blood draw, but still no dialysis," Doctor Lazar explains. "And cut down a bit on the exercise. Thirty-mile bike rides are too much. Six-mile walks are too much. You are running the risk of being dehydrated. That's not good for all the tubes in your kidneys. You don't want them to close down."

You cut back. Two-mile walks (maybe three). Six-mile bike rides (but maybe two or three times a day).

"The rule of thumb is to drink if you're thirsty," the nurse practitioner, Kathleen H. Custer, explains.

You drink more fluids. You can feel your body respond with a slightly better balance, less exhausted. But you also gain four pounds overnight. You think, maybe the kidneys aren't ready to be set free.

After the blood tests, you return to the dialysis center for a consultation with Doctor

Eric and Super Nurse Kathy. The results are not in yet.

They will call you when they are. You bike back home, sneak in an extra six miles.

The call comes around 5:30 PM. The numbers are fantastic.

"We're tap-dancing over here," Kathy Custer says. "Your creatinine level fell to 2.5. All the numbers are in range, except for the ones affected by the steroids." You are silent. "You're probably hyperventilating," she says.

"I can't talk because I'm breathing into this paper bag," you mumble, laughing.

And so you join that rare group of people who have made it back to shore.

You are officially off dialysis, at least for now. You are monitored closely by some of the best and the brightest.

They try to slow you down on your physical assault, saying you are doing too much. But you still cheat a little. The extra mile here. A few more pushups there.

Sargeant Rhyder stands in the background at parade rest. "You did OK, kid. I nev er thought you'd make it through one round. You did OK."

If all goes well, they will remove the chest catheter. You have not been dialyzed for over a week now, after undergoing that debilitating treatment three days a week, almost five hours at a time, for many months.

You feel alright. And thankful for your wife Kerstin's love and caring.

She has not slept well for a long time. She sleeps better now.

You feel humble because of the love of family and friends and the attention of doctors who genuinely care and nurses and dialysis technicians who heroically try to save people every single day. And prayers. And the medicine that works. And an extraordinary doctor who understands how to create an escape route from a devastating disease.

And you thank Sergeant Rhyder. His guardian warrior's spirit has always been there for you.

Semper Fidelis.

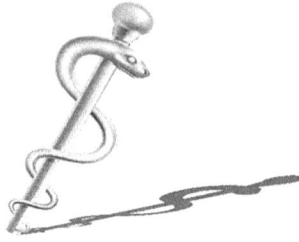

Warrior Patient Rule 12: Exercise and proper diet are essential medicines. If you screw up on food, start again. If you think you cannot do anything physical, wiggle your toes.

Chapter 13

Wraparound Shingles

Rolling over in bed at night is an eye-opening experience.

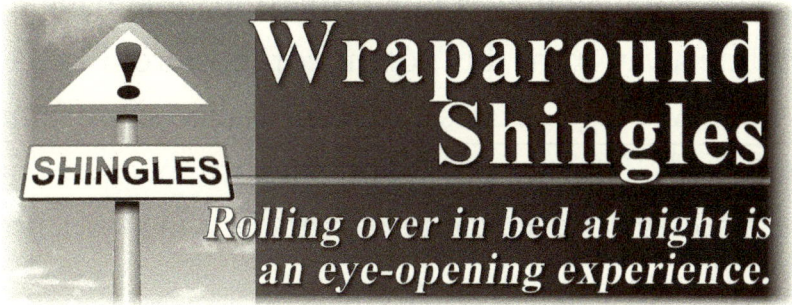

You beat cancer, and you walk away from renal failure on your own two kidneys, although you still have kidney disease. They do not function at 100%. They probably never will. Your relentless battle has scarred them. But they have thrown down their crutches, at least for now.

Doctor Eric Lazar will soon start to wean you off the steroid, prednisone.

Prednisone is a popular wonder drug, fighting everything from asthma to Crohn's disease, from multiple sclerosis to lupus. Physicians use it to prevent rejection during transplants. It's crucial in the treatment of leukemia, Hodgkin's lymphoma, and muscular dystrophy. And it is a critical part of the road map built by Doctor Eric Lazar to let you escape from the cellblock of kidney dialysis.

Prednisone is a powerful drug. You have to tiptoe away from this potent corticosteroid.

At high doses, it can have significant adverse effects on your health because it suppresses the immune system, leaving patients more susceptible to infections.

Stopping prednisone cold turkey is like braking a speeding car by running it into a tree. It works, but it gets a little messy on the inside.

So Doctor Eric Lazar will carefully monitor your withdrawal from prednisone: 60mg, then 40, then 20, then 10, then 5, then 2.5, and finally none at all.

It will take several months, but for now, you continue 60mg every morning, your maximum dosage.

Of course, one disease's escape route can become another's welcoming mat. The massive quantities of prednisone are lovely news for the deadly infection of MRSA. It has not gone away. It hides, takes a vacation, waits.

Before coming off dialysis, the male nurse who administers your iron shots in the center asks: "Did you have chickenpox when you were a kid?"

"Not a clue," you tell him.

He is handing out the morning energy bar, the only part of the kidney dialysis ritual that you enjoy. Of course, the candy bar would never pass dietician Michele's "good foods" test, because it contains chocolate and peanut butter, both of which disappear on a diet for kidney disease. Nobody addresses this issue. Perhaps the dialysis center assumes that patients will not recover, so what's the harm? Maybe they make a profit on the energy bars that builds muscles in their balance sheet. Who cares? The energy bars taste great. You tell all of your friends that the candy bar is the only reason you decided to get kidney disease in the first place.

"Do you want to get a shingle shot?" the candy man asks.

"You bet," you say.

But the next day, Doctor Lazar takes dialysis off your list of medical requirements.

You will never enter the dialysis center again, God willing. You ring the waiting room buzzer, ask about the shingles shot. "Sorry, you're no longer a customer here." That sounds just fine. You can live with that, in every respect.

You do not scratch the shingles shot off your medical "To Do" list. You plan to get it at Walgreens or CVS.

It's a live vaccine given as a single injection, usually in the upper arm.

It does not guarantee you won't get shingles, but it usually works.

As horror stories of the virus spread faster than the virus itself, pharmacies do an increasingly brisk business in shingles shots. Kerstin decides to get her vaccine from her primary physician at the Cleveland Clinic.

You will do it as soon as you're confident that the kidney police won't drag you back into the dialysis center. But your top priority is to get rid of the hole Doctor W. Anthony Lee punched in your chest.

In the pre-op area of the Boca Raton Regional Hospital, the station nurse goes through her usual checklist. Then they wheel you from the prep room into the operating theater.

"Remember me?" you ask Doctor Lee. He shows some teeth in a slight grimace and shakes his head. Catheters. They all look the same.

You point at the two plastic tubes sticking out of your chest.

"I bet you don't take a lot of these out," you say.

"Bad bet," he says. "I have a lot of patients who upgrade to a fistula or graft." The chest catheter was a quick route into dialysis, a way to gain access to the artificial kidney immediately. Later you can move up to the gold standard of a permanent fistula.

"I'm upgrading to nothing," you say. "That's the real gold standard in your line of work, the ultimate upgrade."

"I remember you," he says.

The operation is quick, with a local anesthetic. The doctor performs his surgical magic and carefully withdraws the catheter intact. You get a couple of stitches. You're done. And then you go home, and for the first time in almost four months, you take a shower. You swim. You have a life. Somehow the shingles vaccine disappears from your mind.

A few weeks later, you're drying yourself with a towel after a good swim when the right side of your chest suffers an identity crisis.

It does not know whether to tickle you with a feather or sear your flesh with burning pain. It settles on both.

You've never felt anything like it before in your life. Maybe you were swimming a little too hard, or too long.

It goes away after a while.

You have an appointment with Doctor Donald Heiman, infectious diseases, the next day. Discuss it with him.

When you wake up in the morning, red, blistering alligator scales have attached themselves to the right side of your chest, creeping around to your back.

"Nice," Doctor Heiman says. "Classic shingles." He admires them briefly and then tells you to drop your tennis shirt back into place. The super-light fabric drifts over your skin. It hurts like hell. Now you remember that you forgot to get the shingles shot.

The doctor tells you to bur an over-the-counter medicine at the pharmacy, a white powder you mix with water and apply to the shingles with a paintbrush. It helps. But the ticklish, blistering pain remains, elevated by the slightest movement.

Prednisone is not a culprit in the shingles attack. It can help fight the inflammation, but not the pain. Your weakened immune system and the MRSA infection lurking inside you have probably thrown out a welcome mat to the virus.

Nobody knows what makes shingles rear its ugly red rash.

It develops from the same virus that unleashes chickenpox. If you ever had chickenpox, you can get shingles.

The Centers for Disease Control and Prevention (CDC) suggests that anyone over 40 years old has probably had chickenpox, even if they don't remember it.

According to the CDC, one in three people over the age of 60 will get shingles in their lifetime. Nearly a million Americans sign up for it every year.

None of them volunteers for its agony.

Shingles is a nasty, painful thing. It can spread to your eyes and cause permanent blindness and hearing loss.

You do not touch the shingles when you have them. The alligator blisters eventually break, form small sores, dry and form crusts. In two or three weeks, the crusts fall off.

Usually, there is no scar afterward (not valid in your case). The pain often goes away after two or three months, but not always. It can last a lifetime.

A year after shingles wraps you in its alligator skin, you still hurt. There are no shingles left, of course, although close examination shows a trail of scars circling the right side of your chest. The simple act of putting on a shirt remains uncomfortable. Rolling over in bed at night is still an eye-opening experience.

By now, it has gone beyond the shingles designation. They classify it as post-herpetic neuralgia, a long-lasting nerve pain.

There is no cure for post-herpetic neuralgia, although there are treatment options to ease the symptoms.

"Why does it hurt even when I put on a T-shirt," you ask the doctor.

"It's called allodynia."

The medical world possesses many three- and four-syllable threats.

Medical experts define allodynia as pain on the skin caused by something that usually does not cause pain, like clothing, or a hard stare from Kerstin when you tell her you're going to run around naked for the rest of your life because clothes hurt too much.

Allodynia signals come from specialized nerves that sense information from the top layer of your skin.

Pain caused by touch is called tactile allodynia, suffering from any movement against the skin is called mechanical allodynia, and the agony you feel related to temperature is called thermal allodynia.

You have hit the jackpot.

You have all three.

There are many gimmicky products on the market that promise to fix this. Some legitimate drugs can also work, although the list of their possible side effects suggests that the cure might be worse than the disease for a person with your health profile.

There are also alternative solutions like hypnotherapy and acupuncture. In some states, like Colorado, you can send the problem up in smoke with marijuana.

By now, you are getting smarter about the long list of things that are hurting you.

You are becoming a valid Warrior Patient, a battle-weary veteran, more than willing to fight for every inch of your life. You know what you can and what you cannot fix. You understand what your body has gone through, and what it must still go through.

"The neuralgia will get better over time," doctors say, and you can feel it slowly receding from your body. "It might take years."

"What if I run out of time?" you ask.

"Then it won't matter."

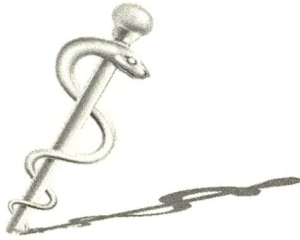

Warrior Patient Rule 13: Do not let today turn into tomorrow's "too late." Get your shingles shot. Get a flu shot. Do not die waiting "just one more day" to visit the doctor.

Chapter 14

A Smiley Face Wearing a Mask

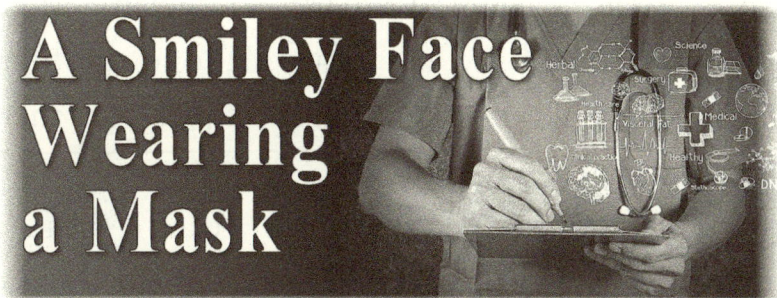

When the journey from medical dope to healthy hope begins, your medical team has one doctor, a Primary Physician.

When it ends, over a dozen (including surgeons) fight for your survival. The team includes two urologists (urinary tract specialists), a nephrologist (kidney specialist), an oncologist (cancer specialist) who is also a hematologist (blood specialist), a cardiologist (heart specialist), an infectious diseases specialist, a neurologist (nervous system specialist), an ophthalmologist (eye specialist), five world-class surgeons, and one excellent home care organization (we dump a bad one).

You choose every one of them carefully, and only one of them is the result of a referral from your original Primary Physician. Most important, they are all aware of one another. They coordinate online with copies of their doctors' notes.

Most (not all) read each other's information and opinions. They keep up to date with a printout of your medical history, which you keep on your computer. It includes all the doctors (with addresses and phone numbers) who contribute to that history. When visiting a doctor's office, they receive the latest information concerning your health, your medications, and any past and future procedures. Equally significant, you understand how each of them helps you, and you know the processes they take.

As a Warrior Patient, you arm yourself with information and a will to survive. You continuously listen to your body for whispers and hints of danger.

You do not fear the danger (well, maybe a little). What you're looking for is a playing field tilted in your favor, where you can fight an unfair fight against the medical problems of life.

Bicycling suddenly gets tough. Daily 20 to 30-mile rides start to make your buttocks sore. A giant gray "sitting donut" slips onto the chair in your second-floor office. Swiveling around in front of computers for more than two hours becomes a noticeable pain in the butt.

You are an equity trader as well as a real estate broker, alone in an office you built just for those purposes. You slide back and forth in your well-cushioned chair, surrounded by five hi-speed computers designed and made into a U-shaped layout. It represents an odd safety zone, with 18 different monitors delivering almost instant information about financial and real estate markets. One bank of monitors is for writing and medical research.

All of this operates as an electronic security blanket. It squeezes knowledge and information out of the world in which you live.

However, your butt hurts a lot. Your first thought is hemorrhoids, which you have never suffered from in your life, but after a few weeks of self-treatment, the growing discomfort suggests something more serious. Going to the bathroom becomes increasingly difficult and painful. MRSA has decided to attack, and it will attempt to kill you, from the bottom up.

You can feel the infection growing in your body. When this becomes obvious, it is almost too late.

The infectious diseases specialist, Doctor Donald F. Heiman, is a very likable person. He's pretty laid back. Honesty keeps tumbling out of his mouth. He does not want to give you any antibiotics such as Vancomycin, which might push your kidneys into a flare-up.

He coordinates closely with Doctor Eric Lazar as you teeter on the tightrope between kidney disease and infection.

There have been no dialysis sessions for almost six weeks.

The numbers remain good. But Doctor Lazar has a warning at every appointment: "A kidney flare-up can occur at any time. You need to continue your maximum daily dose of 60mg of prednisone."

The doctors know the steroids compromise your immune system, but necessarily so.

It is a risk that you must take, and one with which you agree.

At an appointment with Doctor Heiman, you tell him about the pain in your backside. He takes a peek and immediately sends you to Doctor Jose F. Yequez, a colon and rectal surgery specialist at Surgical Associates of Palm Beach County.

Doctor Yequez has completed a Research Fellowship at Jackson Memorial Hospital in Miami, Florida.

He's a colleague of Doctor W. Anthony Lee, who punches a hole in your chest and then repairs it over four months later when you escape from dialysis.

Doctor Yequez is a tough-looking guy, with a voice much softer than his appearance (dark hair, mustache, and goatee). He's likable from the start. In his examination room, you lean your body over a medical bench as he looks at the problem.

"I cannot do anything about this here," he says. "This is very bad."

His voice sounds urgent.

"What is it?" you ask.

"You must go to the hospital. It requires immediate surgery. It is a terrible abscess."

"I can't go to the hospital right now," you say. "I have important business I have to deal with today and tomorrow." The business has quite a few zeros in it.

"You need to go to the hospital," he says. "This is a life-threatening abscess."

"In two days, I can go," you say. "But I can't go right now. It's not going to happen."

You have too much money at stake.

If you die in a hospital without squaring things up, Kerstin might not know what to do.

It will take two days to neutralize any financial danger, and there's no alternative in your mind.

"You need to go to the hospital," he repeats. He stareas into your eyes. "This can kill you. Understand?"

"In two days. I need two days."

He shakes his head. He is upset. He gives you a local anesthetic, calls in his nurse, and performs a temporary drainage operation. It hurts a lot, even with the anesthetic. The sickening odor of death reaches your nostrils from the putrid puss that he squeezes out of the abscess. It will take two days to wrap up this important business, and you cannot think of any way around that fact. You have painted your life into a corner without realizing it.

Leaving the examination room, you apologize to Doctor Yequez: "Sorry for being such a pain in the ass." Neither of you smiles.

"Two days," he says. "You must go immediately to the emergency room."

He sends you back to Doctor Heiman, where an IV of antibiotics (Vancomycin and Invanz) drips through a vein on your wrist, the first antibiotic treatment in many months. It takes an hour and a half. There is no longer a convenient entry port into your heart. The infection, the abscess must be confronted with powerful antibiotics. They repeat the treatment the following day.

You suddenly walk a tightrope stretched taut between your kidneys and your infection. Don't look down.

The abscess on your right butt, Doctor Yequez warns, might lead to gangrene and a putrid open wound, especially in someone with an immune system compromised by prednisone. Those complications might lead to multiple surgeries and the possible need for a colostomy, where a surgeon creates an additional opening in your body for the discharge of human waste. Your brother, Philip, has a good friend who had a colostomy. His friend died before his forty-fifth birthday.

You go on the internet and research what Doctor Yequez has said, look at sickening pictures of people with open wounds into whose footsteps you might stumble. The pictures scare you. Remember Fred, your roommate, when you were last at the Boca Raton Regional Hospital. He fought for his life because of an open wound, although you never saw it. You wonder again whether or not he made it. You start to think of him often.

Your necessary business finally concludes successfully, and Kerstin takes you to the emergency room at the Boca Regional Hospital the next day before the sun rises.

It takes most of the morning to get admitted as you remain in the emergency room area. The doctors and nurses go through a long list of things that might go wrong during the operation or as a result of it. You don't remember receiving such a laundry list of potential complications and risks in any of your other hospitalizations, but you sign the consent papers. The signature looks shaky. You still have not been admitted to the hospital.

In the middle of the afternoon, they finally take you into the pre-op area. You meet Doctor David S. Morse, an anesthesiologist, and Doctor Yequez. Surprisingly, Doctor Heiman appears as well. He will administer IV antibiotics during the operation. Nurses wheel you into the operating theater on your back, and they put compression devices on your legs that tighten and release, tighten, and release. Doctor Morse puts a mask over your face. The compression sequence squeezes your legs two more times before you tumble into a dark hole somewhere in an alternate universe.

They flip the patient's body over and put it in a jack-knife position. Doctor Yequez inspects the abscess cavity and partially drains it with a surgical tool that controls bleeding. The nurse takes cultures. Then Doctor Yequez examines the abscess again and uses a piece of surgical equipment called a Bovie to cut and cauterize an elliptic incision. It encompasses an area larger than the abscess. An ellipse looks like a circle squashed into an oval or two cupped hands put together to hold water. It will be the shape of your initial open wound once the surgery is over. Doctor Yequez uses the Bovie to slice and scoop out the abscess until nothing but healthy tissue remains. Dead, damaged, and infected tissue gets tossed into the red bag. They have to slice down to the muscle in the butt attached to the bone. The Bovie cauterizes the wound and, with the help of a single stitch, all the bleeding stops. Peroxide and saline solutions irrigate your injury, which they pack it with sterile, absorbent gauze.

The entire operation takes 34 minutes. You are unconscious for 40 minutes. Your throat is sore when you wake up because they have to put a breathing tube down it during the procedure.

Doctor Yequez is a great surgeon. The operation is a success.

And the wound is very BIG.

Finally, they admit you to the hospital for evaluation. It will take four days. The IV antibiotic drips continue during this recovery. The tightrope stretched between kidneys and infection remains locked in place.

You have a roommate, and he is also an ex-Marine. You start swapping stories. He is in Korea, at the Inchon Reservoir, a member of what Marines call the Chosin Few, survivors of the Frozen Chosin, part of the 1st Marine Division. It breaks through communist Chinese lines in North Korea in one of the most significant military retreats in history in the early winter of 1950. With other UN troops, the Marines effectively destroy seven Chinese divisions trying to stop their escape to the port of Hungnam. Marine losses numbered 836 killed and 12,000 wounded (mostly frostbite). Precise casualties for the Chinese remain unknown, but estimates are 35,000 killed.

"Only Marines can snatch victory from the jaws of retreat," you tell your roommate, and you both laugh. *Semper Fi.*

You are going to have a good time together during your recovery.

Suddenly nurses and orderlies rush into the room and wheel his bed away, down the hall. You never see him again.

"What's going on?" you ask the nurse. She's wearing a mask.

"Your cultures," she says. "From your operation. You have Mersa." She slaps a red sticker on the door. "You are not allowed out of this room," she says.

Kerstin arrives with my computer and other things from home. "Nice," she says. "You have a whole room to yourself."

"You just have to know the magic word," you tell her. She looks at you.

"Mersa," you say.

"Well, we knew that," she says.

"They didn't," you say, waving towards the nursing station beyond the door with its big red sticker. You tell Kerstin all about the quickest and bravest hospital roommate you ever had.

"So he escaped again," she says. "This time from you." Sometimes Kerstin can be very funny. Every single person who is married to you for forty years gets like this.

The following day, Doctor Steven E. Morris visits. He is covering for your Primary Doctor, Susan Barish. You are admitted to the Boca Raton Regional Hospital by the Hospitalist because nobody can get hold of your primary doctor, and now Personal Physicians Associates is playing catch-up to get on board the gravy train. If they show up, they can bill Medicare for the beautiful job that they are not doing.

In his medical notes, Doctor Morris writes that the patient has renal failure, and it is "clearly worsening." Doctors often make small mistakes in their medical records, but this is a whopper. He has no clue that the patient has escaped from kidney dialysis, and he is getting better, not worse. His report says your mother dies of colon cancer. She beat that disease into complete remission and finally dies of heart failure at the age of 94.

Doctor Steven Morris says your brother has multiple myelomas. You have no idea what this means. He might have multiple personalities, depending on whether he's talking to a woman or a man, but not numerous myelomas. And about which brother is he talking?

Personal Physicians Associates maintains a solid lock on its record of confusion, ignorance, and mediocrity.

Doctor Eric Lazar also visits and sets up continued visits every two weeks once the hospital releases you. The numbers still look good, and he will start to reduce the amount of prednisone you take. Your immune system needs to toughen up.

Doctor Heiman continues treating you with Vancomycin and Invanz.

Your kidneys have not flared up during their reunion with antibiotics.

Another reunion occurs two doors down the hospital corridor. The nurses have removed the red sticker from the door because your MRSA is apparently under control, no longer a threat to people who glance in your direction. You are allowed to wander around the floor, or as one of your irreverent visitors suggests: "Get out there and swing a cheek, Williams. Show them what you got." Somewhat less than you had before.

As you are making your rounds, you notice a redhead in one of the rooms.

"Judy?" you say.

She is a former colleague of Kerstin and yours from your days at Arvida Real Estate (once a powerhouse in the industry, but now gone). You develop and run the Accelerated Sales Division, which sells homes using an Open Bid program (sort of like an auction). Judy is one of Arvida's best real estate agents.

"Temple?" she says. It's the old home week at the Boca Raton Regional Hospital. You are also neighbors at the Boca Country Club, but you never see each other because you live in subdivisions at opposite ends of the community. You run with a different crowd.

"It's about time we all got together," she tells you. "But this is a crummy way to do it." You laugh, and trade wound stories, and you tell her that your doctor has turned you into "a perfect A-hole."

"You always were one," she laughs with gusto, and so do you.

"Actually," Kerstin tells you, "when it's all bandaged up, it looks sort of like a smiley face wearing a mask."

"And when I take the mask off?" you ask. Kerstin frowns. She does not like this part of your journey because it is a big, deep wound.

You go home after four days at the hospital. A home care nurse named Marsha Norris from Home Health Associates comes every day to take your temperature, check your blood pressure, and change and pack your wound. Kerstin likes Marsha a lot because it means Kerstin does not have to pack the injury, which entails irrigating it and then putting a lot of sterile gauze into it. Then you very carefully and gently cover it with bandage strips. Kerstin is an extraordinary partner in your life, a relentless worker, a beautiful woman, and a wonderful wife. She draws the line at stuffing gauze into large open wounds in your butt.

They do not stitch together open wounds like yours. They must heal from the inside out. It is a slow process, and your immune system needs to function well for it to happen.

Doctor Heiman's office continues administering antibiotic IVs. Patients usually fill all three chairs in the treatment area, while a male nurse named Scott entertains us with tales of his Emergency Medical Service (EMS) days.

He has spent a lifetime trying to put the world back together.

He has one "particularly funny story of a motorcycle accident where nobody can find the rider's head." They do know the man is from Norway because they find a passport in his jacket. Nurse Scott calls this story "The Headless Norseman." They eventually find the victim's helmet, which includes his head, in a canal on the side of the road.

Humor in an infectious disease office can have a harsh edge.

The day comes when Nurse Scott administers your last IV treatment. He hands you a Specialists In Infectious Diseases Certificate of Merit. It reads:

Let Be It Declared To All Present That Temple Williams, having completed the prescribed course of antibiotic treatment with a proficiency in the Science & Art of being cheerful, patient, and outstanding in cooperation; is therefore entitled to receive certification as an active member in our Favorite Patients Club; subject to all the rights, honors and privileges thereof.

Donald F. Heiman, MD, signs it. You look in his office on the way out and thank him for all he has done for you. "And, of course, the Certificate of Merit," you say. "But you have to work on the punctuation in the certificate. It has a serious semicolon problem."

You smile at each other. Doctor Heiman has become a valued member of your survival team, and you appreciate his genuine concern and the concern of everyone in his office.

"I never want to see you again," he says.

You laugh. Hopefully, the doctor's wish comes true. The MRSA will probably always be there, but at least now, your immune system has developed some muscle, and the deadly infection is under control.

The wound begins to heal, slowly at first, but then more and more rapidly.

When you take your first shower after coming out of the hospital, the bandage comes off, and the sterile gauze packing drops to the shower floor, nasty, stained, and an awful lot of it. You carefully feel the wound, surprised by its depth and size.

As the injury heals, less and less packing drops to the shower floor. Every morning you peel off the bandage, preparing for Nurse Marsha Norris.

"It's going to take a long time for you to heal," Marsha says when you first meet. You walk a mile that day.

"I am surprised how well this is healing," Marsha says after a week. You are up to three miles.

"I don't think I've ever seen a wound heal this fast," she says a week later.

You do five miles.

"You're not going to need me pretty soon," she says three weeks into the treatment.

"You're done," Marsha Norris says after a month.

"You're a wonderful nurse," you say, every time, meaning it.

Finally, there is light at the end of your long and painful tunnel. Unfortunately, you can't see it very well.

You're going blind.

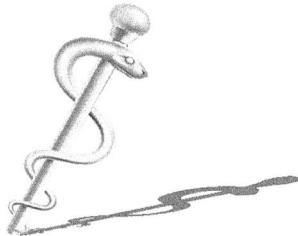

Warrior Patient Rule 14: Save your medical records. Hospitals can give you a CD of your info for a few bucks. You may not understand it all, but it's terrific reading if you have a hard time sleeping.

Chapter 15

The Eyes Have It

Everybody backs away from the diseased cyclops.

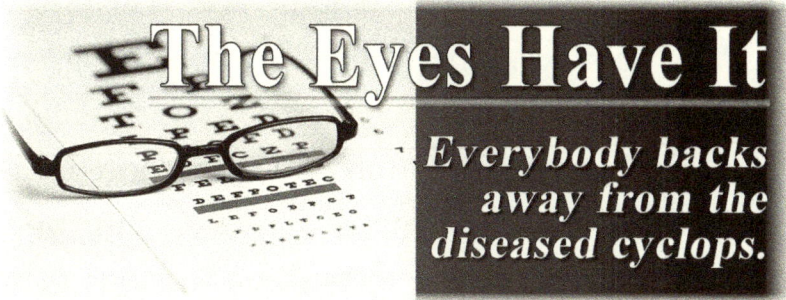

The family's patriarch, Lewis Croxton Williams, dies of complications resulting from Alzheimer's Disease, a terrifying illness that takes twelve years to steal his entire mind. The sickness crumples his body from a 6'2" good-looking man of dignity and dry humor into a fetal ball that remembers nothing and recognizes nobody.

None of his children knows him that well because he does not understand them. He spends a lot of time at the office. Considering the antics and personalities of his children, and their willingness to rule their lives with untethered curiosity, your father's decision to avoid his spawn may be a reasonable one. You learn to love him for his honesty, integrity, intelligence, and wit as you grow older. You and your father become very comfortable with one another as you approach middle age. It happens in many families. The fathers do not change as much as the children.

No one in the family seems to notice his early signs of Alzheimer's Disease. But one, perhaps in retrospect, gets branded on your brain: his eyes.

"Dammit Lyd," he says to your mother, "I can't read the paper. There's something's wrong with my eyes."

His Ben Franklin glasses perch at the end of his nose, useless on the small print in *The Wall Street Journal*. It happens before large type editions exist.

"Have them examined, Lew," she says. And he does. He rattles off the 20/20 line on the optometrist's eye chart with ease and the one below it, too.

Your father repeats this tragic scenario three times, with different eye doctors, before everyone finally realizes he can read the words of a newspaper perfectly, they just never seem to get to his brain cells.

Your mother has a different eye problem in her old age: macular degeneration. She can't see in the center of her vision field because of damage to her retina.

She still has excellent peripheral vision, and the eyes in the back of her head immediately see anything anyone tries to pull off behind her back.

But she has to turn her head to the side to knit, using her peripheral vision.

She loves to knit. Every child's home overflows with rugs and pillowcases with her initials "LEW" (Lydia Emmet Williams) in the corner of each gift.

She particularly enjoys giving you one, bordered with flowers, with a large blue message knit in the middle: "Be reasonable ... Do it my way" (with no period at the end and unnecessary ellipses). You are an editor at The Reader's Digest when she gives you this, an editor who cannot resist telling her that it suffers from a punctuation disorder.

"Read the message, Temple," she says.

Eventually, she must put down her knitting needles, an act of sad, final sacrifice in a life filled with wonder, comfort, intelligence, and laughter. She listens to TV instead of watching it. Talking books put her to sleep at night. Oh, what she would give to fall asleep with a book in her face.

Eyesight is essential in your family, in every family, and you have a familial fear of losing it. You are a writer, a journalist, an editor, all of which require an eyes-on approach to life. When the journey from medical dope to healthy hope begins, your sight is good. But now, your left eye is rapidly approaching legal blindness (20/200).

Your right eye starts to push the dimmer switch lower as well.

It's most notable at night. If you hold a hand over your right eye, your left eye sees the world through a thick gray fog. Night driving becomes a challenge; then, it starts to feel dangerous. Your childhood history of severe car accidents takes away the car keys whenever the sun goes down.

Prednisone probably affects your eyes, an oil slick on the fearful downhill slide into blindness. The wonder drug that saves your kidneys has serious side effects. Among the major ones are blurred vision, cataracts, and glaucoma. Go to the eye doctor. Find out how much trouble you face. It frightens you.

A bike accident puts the skids on plans for an eye examination.

You are biking on a road that leads to the Everglades, Florida's famous River of Grass. It's going to be a long trip, maybe 40 miles, and the speedometer has clocked five of them when a bicycle built for two pulls across the bike path fifty yards away.

The owners are pushing it, not riding it. Two choices: drop down into a very deep rain drainage area or jump the roadside curb and swerve around the young couple standing next to their bicycle built for two.

"Heads up!" you shout. "I'm coming on your left!"

You have chosen to jump the roadside curb rather than search for snakes in the grass at the bottom of the drainage ditch. The young couple does not see you. They are dancing, with their ears plugged into their iPods, and the two-seater stretches entirely across the bike path.

You jerk up on the handlebars to lift the front of the bike higher to swerve around them, but the rear tire skids along the curb, and you slam into the sidewalk. Your leg has a skid mark from the knee to your ankle, and it's bleeding where the skin gets road burned by the cement.

"Are you OK?" the man asks, pulling out his earplugs.

"Bad place to park your bike," you say. "Bad place to dance."

They apologize with happy smiles and ride off. At a CVS pharmacy about three hundred yards down the road, you buy a lot of sterile gauzes, some hydrogen peroxide ("Ouch that hurts"), a topical antibiotic cream, and elastic bandage wraps. The men's room at the pharmacy becomes your triage center. The trip to the Everglades gets canceled. You pedal back home.

The following week you have an eye examination at the Aker Kasten Eye Center. The leg wound is healing quite nicely for a two-and-a-half-foot-long road burn.

You wear shorts to let it breathe. The antibiotic salve rubbed over the scab makes it appear much more threatening and dangerous.

During the check-in for your eye examination, one of the three nurses in the area steps back, points at the road burn, and says: "What's that?"

"That's a bicycle built for two," you say, "on my way to the Everglades on a 40-mile bike trip that never got further than five miles. You see, I had Mersa and ...."

That's as far your storytelling gets. Everybody backs away from the diseased Cyclops. You try to calm things down by telling them that the MRSA is under control.

That's like saying the sticks of dynamite strapped to your leg won't go off unless someone happens to mention them.

You have to leave. Come back when the wound completely heals. Do not come back before then. The exit door is right over there. Out you go.

Two weeks later, guess who's wearing long pants? Nobody recognizes the Cyclops with

MRSA. You go through a complex series of eye tests. The first and most recognizable one is reading the chart. If you can see a series of letters at 20 feet that generally are visible at that distance, you have 20/20 vision. If you can see at 20 feet what an average person can grasp at 40 feet, then you have 20/40 vision.

Your left eye clocks in at 20/180. What a normal eye can see easily at 180 feet, you can only make out when you get within 20 feet.

The left eye is just a blink away from legal blindness.

The right eye registers 20/80.

They put drops in your eyes and run you through a series of multi-syllable tests that measure what's needed to bring them back to standard 20/20 vision (refraction). They shine and slide very bright lights into your eyes to test your pupil function. They test peripheral vision and something called ocular motility, which is way beyond your pay grade of understanding, although it seems related to double vision and brain disorders. Call yourself crazy. You pass the test. They measure the pressure in your eyes and examine your retina with a microscope-powered machine.

"You have absolutely no macular degeneration," the doctor says.

"Are things that I see getting through to my brain?" you ask. The doctor looks at you sideways. "My father had Alzheimer's, and he could read things, but after a while, he could not understand them."

"You're fine as far as I can see, as far as you can see, too," the doctor says.

Two enormous sighs of relief.

You do not want to follow in the visual footsteps of your parents.

You do have cataracts, a real humdinger in your left eye. You schedule surgery. The surgeon will be Doctor Jill F. Rodila, educated at Wheaton College and the University of Illinois College of Medicine.

You do not tell her you are an Ohio State fan. You never know with these Illinois people. Doctor Rodila looks like she comes from good Midwestern stock, reddish-brown hair, healthy complexion, determination in her eyes, and confidence in her abilities. You can trust her with your vision.

First, they will do the almost-blind eye, and then a week later, they will do the not-so-bad eye. Because MRSA still lurks in your body, you are probably taking a risk with the eye operation. You do not talk to the people at the Aker Kasten Eye Center about any of this.

Every time you check into a medical facility, you now bring updated sheets of paper that are titled: Doctors & CareGivers, Current Medications, and Medical History.

When you hand them your Medical History sheet, it does mention your continuing problems with MRSA.

You give it to them and hope they don't read it. You need to get your eyes back.

A few days before the surgery, Aker Kasten phones and puts the operation off.

"Why," you ask, convinced that the MRSA police have busted you.

"Doctor Rodila's daughter broke her nose, and we have to reschedule the surgery for a week from now," the nurse says. You catch the word "good" just before it can escape from your mouth. "No problem," you say.

A cataract is a clouding of the lens inside your eye, which causes vision loss. You cannot correct it with glasses, contact lenses, or refractive surgery like LASIK.

At least 20 million Americans over the age of 40 have cataracts in one or both eyes. The procedure removes your existing lens and replaces it with a new artificial one.

You can choose expensive lenses or not-so-expensive ones. Doctor Rodila tells you to get the less costly ones. Doctor Rodila jumps a few rungs higher on the excellent physician ladder.

It's an outpatient procedure. A nurse gives you some delightful happy juice, and you lay on your back in the operating theater. Doctor Rodila is in green scrubs, along with several other people. There is some soothing music going on in the background.

First, she says a prayer, asking God to guide her hands and bring the patient in for a safe landing. It might seem a bit awkward to some people, but think back to the prayers God answered with a "yes" during the fight to get off kidney dialysis.

You are perfectly willing to put your surgeon's fingertips in the hands of God.

They place a sterile drape around your eye. Doctor Rodila makes a tiny incision at the outermost edge of the cornea (the eye surrounding your pupil, which is brown, Kerstin's is hazel). The slice is less than an eighth of an inch. Everyone seems to be having a pretty good time. They are chattering about things and laughing just beyond your comprehension. It is a happy medical team, working well together.

Then Doctor Rodila picks up a large, rusty machete about two feet long. No, just kidding, calm down.

The little hole at the edge of the cornea is just large enough to accommodate a microsurgical instrument about the size of the tip of a pen. It uses ultrasound to break up the cataract, which is then carefully and completely sucked out. Then Doctor Rodila slips in a new artificial lens, tailored to your specific needs by all the eye tests they have run before the surgery.

Doctor Rodila puts a few antibiotic drops in the eye, and the operation is over in about 15 minutes. Nurses wheel you downstairs from the operating theater, and Kerstin is waiting near the entrance to the building.

"Wow," you say. "So, that's what you look like."

"Stop it."

"You look so ... I don't know, Swedish," you say. "I mean, you have blonde hair. I thought you were a brunette. And you have smooth skin, and — ."

"I'm going to get the car," she says to the person handling the wheelchair.

You tell your handler she can leave you there, go back inside. "If I wander off," you say, "she'd probably want you to let go of me."

She tightens her grip on the wheelchair.

You laugh.

You're having fun, and Kerstin is your soul mate. The colors you can suddenly see are unbelievable. You did not know the sky was that blue, and you had no idea palm trees were so green. Everything remains blurred because of the eye drops they have given you, but the brightness of all the colors amaze you.

Doctor Rodila does the other eye a week later. You have a series of appointments to check your vision over the next few months, but the result is 20/20 in both eyes, and the rebirth of vivid colors forgotten years ago.

"I still need reading glasses," you tell Doctor Rodila, "but you told me beforehand that might be the case."

Now the end of your healing journey approaches. The steroid Prednisone has vanished from your medication list. Doctor Eric Lazar has slowly weaned it down from 60 mg to none. Dialysis has not invaded your life for over half a year. Blood tests show that the creatinine level steadily drops to 1.6 (from 5.5 when you had renal failure). The 1.6 is still higher than usual, and it may be the baseline for the rest of your life. But at least now you have a life.

A technician takes a CT scan of your abdomen and pelvis at the Boca Raton Regional Hospital. The abdomen scan shows no kidney stones, no urinary obstruction, and no kidney inflammation. Your liver, spleen, pancreas, and adrenal glands are healthy.

It is an outstanding report.

The pelvis scan shows that the bladder is fine, no longer distended. The human factory is repairing itself. But there is a worsening of the left inguinal hernia. It now contains a loop of the large intestine. A hernia operation represents the final link in your journey from medical dope to healthy hope.

Best of all, the finish line is now visible, clear, and filled with bright colors.

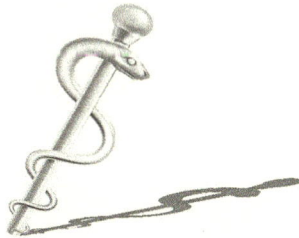

Warrior Patient Rule 15: When a medical facility asks you for your list of medications, add a list of all your doctors and medical procedures as well. If they say they don't need them, consider treatment elsewhere.

Chapter 16

The Imaginary Operation

"... here's the good news," he said. "I perform the surgery. They don't."

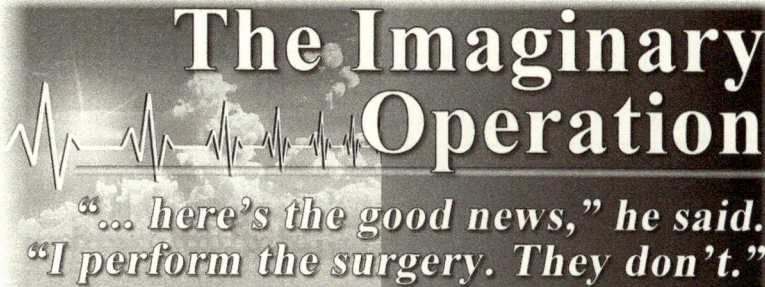

Doctor Matthew A. Klein, a well-tanned surgeon, specializing in hernia operations, motions towards the examination table. "Can you get up on that?"

"I just biked from the dialysis center," you say. "No problem."

Doctor Eric Lazar speaks highly of this surgeon and wants him to take a look at the hernia on the left side of your groin.

Doctor Klein looks like a golfer, probably with a low handicap. Good-looking, lean, maybe a jogger as well. A picture of health. Sliding up on his examination table, you try to make it look as simple as possible. Don't look sick. Let your athletic past reveal itself in the simple act of lifting your body onto an examination bench. Good health screams for attention, bonding, communication. Doctor Klein reads your mind, a bit strange (the event, not your brain cells).

"When Doctor Lazar said he was sending you over, I had no idea how vibrant you'd be," he says.

Even if everyone else sees a down-in-the-dumps dialysis patient, trudging slowly towards a dismal end, this medical professional sees a spark of health, hope, life.

"I feel pretty good," you lie, not feeling all that good.

"Let's take a look at the hernia." He feels the lump. "Nice inguinal hernia."

It hurts a little as he pushes it around. "Doctor Lazar has you on Prednisone," he says. "How much are you taking?"

"A lot. Sixty milligrams. Every day."

The doctor's face assumes his best decision-making mode. He compresses his lips into a thin line and strokes his chiseled chin.

This guy is a pro.

"I don't want to operate on you until you're off the steroids," he finally says.

He will not operate on you just for the sake of performing surgery. He will not treat you as a revenue stream.

You have a flashback to Kerstin's fibroid problem, her nightmare with the false alarm of ovarian cancer.

Doctor Matthew Klein will become your end game, the final link back to health. Almost a year will pass before you meet again.

During that time, the hernia doubles in size. Each night, before falling asleep, you shove it back into your body, squirming a bit until it slips into place behind the sheet muscle of the lower abdomen. Sometimes it slides into place easily. Sometimes it doesn't.

But always, when sleep comes, your intestines are back where they belong, behind the sheet muscle of your abdomen.

Leg lifts try to kick strength back into your stomach muscles every morning. Perhaps these simple exercises can make the hernia disappear. Wake in the morning, twenty leg lifts, slip carefully out of bed, tighten the stomach, stroll into the bathroom with flat, tight muscles.

You look in the mirror, reach for a toothbrush, and, plop; the bulge pops out.

Every day starts with this physical defeat. Hernia belts can keep the bulge within the abdomen wall, but this has no appeal. The problem demands a solution, not a cover-up.

Hernias develop when too much strain pushes part of the intestine through a weak area of the abdominal muscle. Inguinal hernias such as yours appear in the groin area. You have only seen one other hernia in your life.

That occurs decades earlier, at Montefiore Hospital in New York, sticking out of the stomach of a patient in the bed next to you. You have just had your gallbladder removed, and you remain in a fog of anesthesia.

"Can I have your gallstone?" your hospital roommate asks. A small, clear plastic tube next to the bed holds what looks like a tiny brown soccer ball with yellow markings, between a third and a half an inch across. The surgeon has promised to give you any gallstone he removes during the operation. It stands in the shadow of a huge fruit basket from friends.

"I collect gallstones," your roommate says. "Can I have it?"

"Nope. No way," you grunt, painfully, a child protecting a cherished toy. It takes a while for what he says to sink in.

"Why do you collect gallstones?"

"I work in the morgue," he explains. It makes perfect sense to him. It takes a while for you to figure it out.

The autopsy table is a breeding ground for gallstone collectors.

"I've gone through a lot of pain to get this," you say, reaching for the tube holding a small gallstone. "I want to keep it."

He seems disappointed.

"It's a nice color," he tells you.

He can have a banana, an orange, or an apple from my fruit basket. But not the gallstone. He is a tough-looking black person lying on his bed with his upper torso exposed to the waist. "Why do you have a fingertip growing out of your stomach?" you ask him.

He laughs, but with a dismissive snort instead of a smile. "It's an umbilical hernia," he explains to the medical idiot who, like it or not, remains the Official Owner of his Gallstone. You are not bonding very well.

Later that night, however, he is bonding exceptionally well with his girlfriend. She has somehow slipped past the standard visiting hours and into his bed. You are in a great deal of pain at this point. It is the bad old days of gallbladder removal when they draw a scalpel halfway across your abdomen to get a grip on the offending organ. Today they can remove it with non-invasive surgery. But in the early 1980s, they slice and dice you, and it hurts. The commotion in the bed next to you has your nerves on alert. Then it gets much worse.

The door opens, and another woman walks in. It is not your roommate's girlfriend. It is his wife. The room suddenly turns into a wrestling match. Someone bangs into your bed. A large woman stumbles back and sits on your feet. Pain shoots up your body, into your brain, passes down your right arm, and reaches your thumb, which machine guns rapid-fire on the Call Button. Suddenly all the lights go on. The room fills with nurses, doctors, assistants, and four-letter words. When things finally settle down, the gallstone collector has been wheeled away, still in his bed. People shouting continues in the hallway, but it fades into some beautiful new painkillers you have just been given. That is your only experience with hernias until you get one yourself over thirty years later.

On July 17th, you have a pre-op session with a nurse at the Boca Raton Regional Hospital. You review special food and hygiene requirements for the hernia operation, scheduled for July 19th with Doctor Klein.

It's no food or water after midnight and special washing instructions with a super antibacterial soap the night before and the morning of the surgery. Use the super soap below the neck. Avoid the groin area. Not on your face. It can destroy your brand new eyes.

Wash with the soap for five minutes. Then rinse and pat yourself dry. There's no drinking in the morning. No coffee. No juice. No water. Not a drop. Show up at the hospital at 7:15 AM on June 19th with nothing of value. Leave the wallet and jewelry at home. No wedding bands. No cell phones. Wear clean clothes. Who shows up for a hernia operation wearing dirty clothes?

Kerstin drops you off at 7:05 a.m. The nurse at the pre-op session has explained that the procedure might take about an hour. The recovery might last 4 hours.

So Kerstin will probably pick you up around noon and take you back home. No hospital stay is required. The less time you spend in hospitals, the better, because of your MRSA infection, even though it's under control. Hospitals are notorious germ factories.

You and Kerstin tell each other everything will be fine. She drives off.

They'll call her after they wheel you into the recovery area.

"I have surgery at 7:15," you tell the receptionist at the main entrance.

"Last name?"

"Williams."

"Date of birth?"

"Eleven Ten Forty-Two," you answer, followed by your usual lame joke of "too long ago." It receives the usual tired smile. In the medical system, November 10th, 1942, has become an identity more significant than your name.

"11-10-42" sews every medical event of your life together.

The receptionist shuffles through patients' paper piled on her desk.

"Your doctor's name?" she asks, reaching the bottom of the pile.

"Doctor Klein," you answer.

"Which Doctor Klein?"

"Doctor Matthew Klein," you reply. "Surgical Associates."

She shuffles through the paper again. She looks up at you and says: "I think you must be scheduled down the street at the Glades …."

I don't think so," you interrupt. "I had the pre-op right here two days ago with a nurse. Right over there, through those large double doors just off the corridor."

You point at the doors.

The receptionist shuffles through the paper again. No luck. She starts tapping on her keypad, watching the monitor in front of her. Her name is Ingrid, but her dark hair and complexion contain no hint of that common Scandinavian name. She says something in Spanish to another surgical check-in and then turns back to the computer monitor.

"What is your date of birth?" she asks again. Repeat it, minus the lame joke.

She needs your first name. Then she is on the phone with someone. Have a seat. She tells the person on the phone that the patient has an account at the Boca Regional Hospital. Then you are out of earshot, sitting on a bench in reception, watching a silent movie unfold in front of your eyes. The receptionist's mouth moves as she speaks into the phone for several minutes. She hangs up and calls someone else. It takes time, and she handles several other patients between phone calls.

Ingrid finally signals to you. She says: "The doctor canceled your surgery two days ago. The doctor should have called you."

"He did not." Move to the side as she deals with a new patient who has just entered the hospital and requires a wheelchair. They quickly admit the new patient, which somehow creates a warped sense of jealousy in you.

"What am I supposed to do?" you ask. "I was scheduled for surgery. Now. Today."

A sudden wave of hopelessness washes over you.

You have no wallet, no identity, no money, no house keys, and no phone. You are, however, wearing clean clothes.

"Your doctor canceled your surgery," Ingrid repeats. She is not harsh. She has no answer, no solution, and no blame. "He should have called you when he canceled it."

There have been no messages left on the phone answering service and none on either of the cell phones. None appears on the automatic system that kicks in if you are using your home phone and someone calls. No e-mails. You return to the bench and consider walking over to the building where Surgical Associates has its office. It's less than half a mile away.

Let Doctor Klein explain the cancelation himself. But his office will not open for at least another hour.

You left home in a hurry, flustering Kerstin. She forgot her cell phone in your rush to surgery. She will be home soon. She can drive back down to the hospital, pick you up, and you can go over to Surgical Associates to solve this unexpected stupidity together.

You look at the receptionist, smile, and say: "You know they tell you to show up for surgery with nothing but clean clothes on your body. I have no money, no identity, no wedding band, no cell phone. I have nothing with me."

Ingrid listens to this with a concerned forehead. She points to a white Call-A-Taxi phone on the shelf in front of you. "Dial 'nine' first," she says, "and then any local number."

For the next hour, you call home and then Kerstin's cell phone. Space the calls ten minutes apart. No answer. Another ten minutes. No answer. Walk outside into the morning heat. It looks like rain is coming. Another ten minutes. No answer. Back to the reception area. Sit on the hard wooden bench that nobody ever has to use. You go back to the Taxi phone. No answer. Leave increasingly sad messages.

Consider walking home. It's about ten miles. Go along the Boca Rio Trail most of the way, a pleasant bike ride, but a long walk. You have not eaten anything or had a drink for 15 hours, and you feel a little weak in the muggy Florida morning. Storm clouds threaten rain. The walk seems impossible. When Kerstin gets your messages, she will return to the main entrance of the hospital. If you are not there, her imagination will build frightening scenarios. Walking home will take over three hours.

Return to the hospital reception area. Phone again. No answer.

"Can I get you some coffee?" Ingrid asks. "Some orange juice?"

"Special diet," you say. "I was a dialysis patient. Kidneys. Shingles. Abscesses. I have Mersa ...." Your voice trails off like some lost, pitiful child. "Thanks."

Retreat to the bench, humiliated by the situation, and your pathetic attitude.

Ingrid gets up and leaves the area. She comes back a few minutes later and hands you some brownish slips of paper.

"That's five Boca Bucks," she tells you. "There's a cafeteria right around the corner. Charles, can you show Mr. Williams where the cafeteria is, please?"

A young man in blue scrubs guides you there. You sit in the cafeteria and think about people who live on food stamps, and about politicians who want to take food stamps away from them.

A banana, Cheerios, and a medium coffee sneak under your five Boca Bucks. The bitter taste of empathy fills your stomach.

"Thank you for your kindness," you say to Ingrid when you return to the reception area. Try the phone again. Your heart leaps as Kerstin answers, saying she is on her way to the hospital. She has been working out in the gym.

You drive three minutes to the offices of Surgical Associates. The large area on the third floor of the building has just a few people waiting. The receptionist greets you cheerfully, and you tell her that, no, it is not a good morning.

You need to speak to Doctor Klein, who was supposed to meet you in surgery earlier. "Only they told me at the hospital that he canceled the surgery two days ago."

"Doctor Klein is not in," she answers. She almost adds that he is in surgery, but she opens and closes her mouth and says nothing.

"Then we need to speak to his nurse," you tell the receptionist.

"Just a moment," she says. She disappears into the offices of Doctor Matthew A. Klein, returns in a few moments, and says his nurse will be right out to speak to you. You wait. And wait.

You look at the receptionist and are about to say something when she scampers back into the inner sanctum of Doctor Klein. Through the closed frosted glass of his outer office, shadow bodies are moving around.

One shadow hints at a telephone in someone's hand. After a few minutes, the receptionist returns and says the nurse will be right out. Nervously, she admits that someone in his office is trying to phone Doctor Klein's nurse for information.

"So she must be in surgery with Doctor Klein," you smile. "Right?" She repeats that someone will be out in a moment.

Five minutes later, an assistant walks out of the double doors leading to Doctor Klein's offices. "Are you Mr. Williams?" she asks politely. You start to talk, and Kerstin joins the group. Your voice gets a little louder, and the assistant pulls you away from the almost-empty waiting room into a hallway.

She has no answers. She does admit that it was Doctor Klein who canceled the operation, two days earlier, the same day you had the Pre-op meeting with a nurse through the double doors at the Boca Regional Hospital.

"You tested positive for MRSA," the assistant says.

"I have had MRSA for over a year," you answer. "I will probably have it for the rest of my life. Eventually, it might kill me. Doctor Klein knows I have it. All the paperwork I have given to your office mentions it. It may even be one of the reasons I have a hernia. It is not the patient's fault. It is not the fault of an infection. It is a complete screw-up."

"Mr. Williams, I don't know what to say," she says. She pleads that she is the messenger and powerless to answer your questions.

You do not apologize to her. At the start of your journey from medical dope to healthy hope, you might have done so. But not now. "Someone should have at least phoned me about the canceled surgery before I went through all the preparation for it."

"The hospital should have called you," she immediately says.

"That's funny," you answer. "The hospital says the doctor should have called me. Doctor Klein canceled the operation. I showed up. He did not."

She stares at me, and she has nothing left to say. Answers remain far above her pay grade.

"Someone needs to explain this to us."

She nods. She says she will have someone call that afternoon, at the latest.

"I promise," she says.

Later that afternoon, a phone call to Doctor Klein's office gets no further than another promise from an assistant who says that someone will phone before the day is over.

The only telephone calls received are from friends who are surprised at how great you sound after the surgery. You laugh and explain that it was the most uncomplicated surgery in the entire history of medicine because it never occurs. You show up, but the doctor does not.

The offices close at Surgical Associates. Nobody has called. At six p.m., you and Kerstin bicycle down to the tennis courts. You are more aggressive than usual and beat Kerstin, six to two. You quit after just one set and return home. No one has phoned.

Trust is a necessary bond between patient and doctor. With Doctor Matthew A. Klein of Surgical Associates, arrogance and the abusive silence and excuses of his nurse and his assistants shatter that trust.

Will you let Doctor Klein within the scalpel's distance of your hernia? Should you? You no longer trust him, and you do not believe his office. But you need an explanation. Why was the surgery canceled? Why didn't the patient know about it?

The weekend has arrived. You will phone Surgical Associates on Monday, but with a plan: a Warrior Patient's plan.

You spend the weekend and part of Monday writing some of what appears in this chapter. You wait to see if anyone from Surgical Associates will phone. Nobody does. Early on Tuesday morning, you format everything into book pages. Two copies. One for Doctor Klein, one for the hospital.

Temple's imaginary hernia operation

On July 17th, I had a pre-op session with a nurse at the Boca Raton Regional Hospital. We reviewed special food and hygiene requirements for the hernia operation, scheduled for July 19th with Doctor Klein.

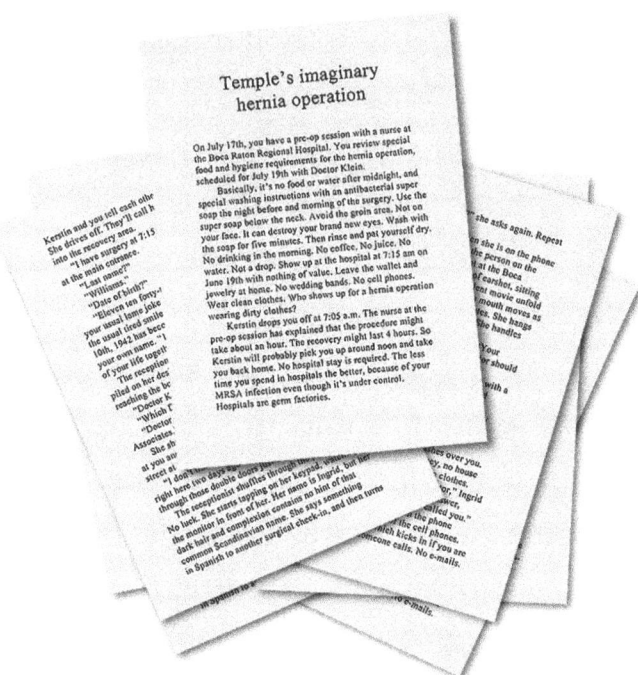

Temple's imaginary hernia operation

On July 17th, you have a pre-op session with a nurse at the Boca Raton Regional Hospital. You review special food and hygiene requirements for the hernia operation, scheduled for July 19th with Doctor Klein.

Basically, it's no food or water after midnight, and special washing instructions with an antibacterial super soap the night before and morning of the surgery. Use the super soap below the neck. Avoid the groin area. Not on your face. It can destroy your brand new eyes. Wash with the soap for five minutes. Then rinse and pat yourself dry. No drinking in the morning. No coffee. No juice. No water. Not a drop. Show up at the hospital at 7:15 am on June 19th with nothing of value. Leave the wallet and jewelry at home. No wedding bands. No cell phones. Wear clean clothes. Who shows up for a hernia operation wearing dirty clothes?

Kerstin drops you off at 7:05 a.m. The nurse at the pre-op session has explained that the procedure might take about an hour. The recovery might last 4 hours. So Kerstin will probably pick you up around noon and take you back home. No hospital stay is required. The less time you spend in hospitals the better, because of your MRSA infection even though it's under control. Hospitals are germ factories.

It ends: **"The weekend has arrived. I will phone Surgical Associates again next week, but I am looking for a new surgeon I can trust —** *To be continued ."*

On Tuesday morning, the waiting room of Surgical Associates has its usual patient count.

Possible patients fill less than a quarter of the fifty or so seats available.

"Please make sure this is given to Doctor Klein," you tell the receptionist. She takes the large white envelope with your address label in the upper left-hand corner. Doctor Mathew A. Klein's name appears very large above DELIVERED BY HAND and PERSONAL. She promises he will get it.

You take a similar envelope over to the Boca Regional Hospital and leave it at their intake area. Then you go back home. Sit down in front of the computer. Keep searching for a new surgeon. You find out where they went to medical school and read their patient comments. You check other sources — the phone rings.

"I want to apologize," Doctor Klein says. His voice rapidly fires each sentence. "I don't even know where to begin. You wouldn't believe what happened. I can't understand it myself. It was just a total —." his voice hangs in the air. You finish it.

"FUBAR," you say. It's an old Navy acronym for Fouled Up Beyond All Recognition. "Fouled" is interchangeable with other words that begin with the letter "F."

Offhand, you can only think of one.

"Screw up," he corrects you. "You wouldn't believe what happened if I told you."

"I might. Tell me what happened."

He does not go anywhere with this. He has not thought things through before calling me. He's a very skilled surgeon, perhaps a brilliant one, but unexpectedly on the wrong end of a conversation. You picture him as a cowboy firing a pistol from his hip, a professional sharpshooter, but too far away from the target.

"I don't want to be the bad guy in your book," Doctor Klein finally says, with authority, not with fear or even sincerity. You decide to remain silent.

"Listen," Doctor Klein says. "I don't know what happened yet, or why, but we can reschedule your operation whenever you want. You tell me when."

You say nothing.

You think about a lawyer admonishing a new intern in his office: "Whatever you do, never ask a witness a question to which you do not know the answer."

"Or I can suggest another surgeon if that's what you want," Doctor Klein suddenly adds. "Whatever you want."

It is an awkward conversation for Doctor Klein, and you can feel it. The weight of the phone in your hand grows heavier.

"A lot of people have told me you're a great surgeon," you finally tell him. "People I trust and respect." The conversation relaxes, but only a little.

"I am," he admits.

You think of the great Hall of Fame baseball pitcher, Dizzy Dean, who said: "It ain't bragging if you can do it." You remember Satchel Paige, The Kid From Cleveland (a movie about him, and the town where you were born and raised). Hall of Fame pitcher Satchel Paige said: "Mother always told me, if you tell a lie, always rehearse it. If it don't sound good to you, it won't sound good to no one else."

When you are a teenager, your father tries to teach you to "count to ten" before saying anything. He recognized impatience as one of your many flaws. Words travel from your vocal cords to your mouth without stopping for a chat with your brain. But you could never get to "ten," so you taught yourself to think of other things: cowboys firing from the hip, lawyers admonishing interns, great athletes explaining lies, and bragging rights.

"My problem is that I don't trust your office," you tell Dr. Klein. "They screwed up the scheduling, and, as your patient, I paid the price. You're only as good as the people that work for you. They *are* you."

"Yeah, well, here's the good news," he answers, dismissing your perceived arrogance a little too quickly. "I perform the operation. They don't."

It is an intelligent statement, and you immediately realize he has probably said it before, to other patients, perhaps too often. You think, "I am not your first *no show*."

"Call my office to reschedule, if you want," Doctor Klein says. "And again, I apologize." The conversation ends.

Think back to when you first meet Doctor Klein. You like him because he does not want to operate on you right away.

He does not treat you like a guinea pig or a revenue stream. The doctor you trust more than any other — Doctor Eric Lazar — says Doctor Klein is an excellent surgeon.

One of Doctor Klein's associates, Doctor Jose F. Yequez, who operates on your abscess, says nothing but good things about him.

You ask Doctor Yequez, during a visit to the Surgical Associates' office six months earlier, if he does hernia operations.

He does.

But during that visit, when you suggest he might want to take a crack at your hernia, he defers to Doctor Klein.

Perhaps it is a professional courtesy, but he has high praise for Doctor Klein.

Kerstin tells you: "You have to start all over if you use another surgeon. You've made your point."

Of course, she's right. It's one of her serious faults.

Two weeks later, Doctor Klein comes to the pre-op room at Boca Regional Hospital. You've been prepped, talked to the anesthesiologist, and everything is good to go.

"Glad you could stop by," you say.

"You wouldn't believe what happened. I can't understand it myself," the doctor repeats from your conversation two weeks earlier.

"It doesn't matter," you tell him, smiling. "Do great work."

And he does.

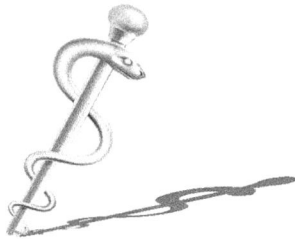

Warrior Patient Rule 16: Make sure all your doctors understand that their reputations depend on how their staff and office operate, and not just on how *they* operate.

Chapter 17

How to count to 9½

You know something bad has happened, but you're afraid to look down at your hand.

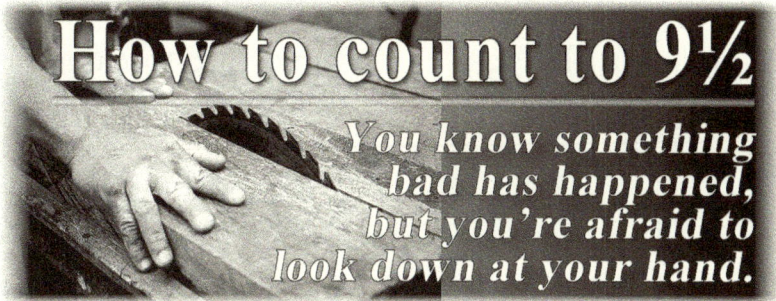

When you are eight years old, your father tells you that you cannot do everything you want to do in life.

"Why not?" you ask.

"Because there are limitations in life."

"Why?"

"Because you cannot do everything you want to do."

"Why not?"

Your mother has just thrown you out of the house. Your father has had to return home from work early to establish your banishment. You are standing next to a large garbage can filled with snakes.

You start with just a single snake, about six feet long, on your bed. Your mother hears you squealing happily in your room and immediately recognizes this as a possible life-threatening situation. She steps into your room and starts to scream.

The beautiful black snake you have brought home is having babies, lots and lots of babies. They squirt out of an opening on her scaled yellow bottom in small translucent sacks, and she bites each one, and babies squiggle out. They are all over your bed, miniature duplicates of Momma Snake.

It may be the best thing that has ever happened to you in your life. You have a snake factory in your room, and you can sell them to your friends for at least a nickel each. That buys a lot of licorice, your favorite candy. At the age of eight, you have become the world's leading snake entrepreneur. Provided, of course, you can get your mother to stop screaming and shouting at you.

You spend much of your life trying to prove that your father's Limitations Ultimatum is entirely wrong. You are a writer, a cop, a Marine, a software developer, a copywriter, an art director, a tree surgeon, a carpenter, a roofer, a welder, an electrician, a plumber, a flooring specialist, a kitchen and bathroom designer, a real estate broker, a statistician, a website developer, a creative director, an editor, a correspondent, a business owner and, briefly, the world's Number One snake entrepreneur (you try to be the top Turtle Entrepreneur a few months later, but that doesn't work out any better than the snake selling business).

"In other words," your friends tell you, "you just can't hold down a job for very long."

Friends like to keep your feet on the ground, but it's been a lot of fun trying to prove your father wrong.

You have recovered very well from all your medical problems although you have a scare at your hematologist's office. They draw blood from you whenever you have an appointment to see Doctor Harold Richter. The Center for Hematology-Oncology, where he works, has its on-site lab analyze it.

Doctor Richter has a calm personality and a no-nonsense approach to medicine. He's the ultimate straight shooter, and you like him. He has been saving the life of an excellent friend of yours for several years.

He's a nice-looking guy who moves deliberately and quickly.

He interns at the VA hospital in New York in the 1980s after graduating from SUNY Upstate Medical University in Syracuse in 1982.

VA hospitals give doctors nerves of steel. They see everything, and they do everything.

You're sitting in an examination room, with your shirt open (nurse's orders), thumbing through some sports magazines.

Doctor Richter rushes in, moving fast. He looks at you with piercing eyes.

"How do you feel!"

It's not a question; it's an exclamation.

"I was fine until you jumped through the door," you say.

You feel your eyes widen.

Something is wrong.

"You're scaring the crap out of me."

He sits down at the computer and kicks up your blood test, which you are pretty sure he has already seen.

"Are you tired?" he asks.

"Not a bit," you say. "I am now wide awake, although I bet my blood pressure is creeping up a few notches. It's probably through the roof right now."

He comes over and pushes and prods you, feels your neck, stethoscopes you front and back, "deep breath, hold it, let it out. Take another deep breath."

He asks you if you have any pain, are you eating well, and the right foods?

"I feel pretty good," you say. And you do.

He sits back down at the computer and tells it: "I don't understand this." He turns to you. "You look good," he says.

"What does the computer say?" you ask.

"We need to do your blood test again."

The computer tells him you are either on your last leg or already dead.

You return to the testing area, get needled again, and return to the examination room.

Doctor Richter comes in as soon as he sees the results.

"You're fine," he tells you.

You don't ask him whose blood it was that he was looking at, but you check for bodies in the men's room and the lobby before leaving the building.

You and Kerstin make up stories about this event. Some poor guy goes home with your blood reports and tells his wife about his miraculous recovery. His wife hugs him, and he drops dead.

You smile about it, but not too much.

Kerstin brings out a new and improved "To Do" list to keep you out of trouble. You enjoy being her favorite handyman. "Fix the patio" tops the list.

You are in the back of the house in Boca Raton, lifting patio screening on a cement slab with a two-ton jack so you can realign the screens and slip drainage holes under it for runoff water. You are cutting three-inch plastic tubing, which you will set in cement under the raised screens.

You have put a new metal cutting blade in your portable table saw. You are on the sixth and final slice of three-inch plastic tubing when the saw blade suddenly grabs you. You jump back from the high-pitched sound of the machine, knowing that something terrible has happened. You look down at your left hand, and the end of your index finger is missing. It's a perfect slice right through the top knuckle. Your first thought comes from curiosity: "So that's how a finger works." Three blood vessels stare at you out of a white bone. The hot saw blade appears to have cauterized them correctly, and there's minimal bleeding. You wonder, briefly, if it will form a scab and heal if you just bandage it up. Then the pain hits.

"Kerstin," you shout, stepping into the courtyard, "we have to go to the hospital. I've cut my finger off." She immediately gets into emergency mode, with which you keep giving her practice: calm, logical, heading for the car, no questions asked. Let's go.

"Wait," you say. "I have to find the finger." It takes a while, but you discover it in the grass six feet from the table saw, lodged in the tip of the orange work gloves you are using. You put it on ice in a plastic container, and you head for the emergency room at the Boca Raton Regional Hospital.

It's Saturday evening, and the ER is not busy at all.

They get hold of Doctor Brandon J. Luskin, an orthopedic hand surgeon, and he makes it to the Emergency Room within twenty minutes. God keeps looking after you, even when you're stupid.

Kerstin says Doctor Luskin is extremely good-looking, maybe even a medical rock star. He comes in dressed casually, and he quickly organizes a team for an operation on your hand. There's almost a party atmosphere surrounding him, filled with excitement and magic.

A lot of people want to work with Doctor Luskin. He has the charisma of a leader, and you can feel it.

"Nice job," he says, looking at your finger. You talk, and you tell him about your medical history. He will make sure you get happy juice that won't damage your kidneys. He will try to keep you out of the hospital after the operation.

"Can you re-attach the finger?" you ask. The doctor doesn't think so. The saw blade chewed up a lot of your knucklebone.

"I was in demolition in Africa," you tell him. "I taught a lot of guys in Mozambique how to blow stuff up. I like to show people I still have ten fingers, proof of how good I was at my job. I guess I can't do that anymore."

"How did the guys you were teaching turn out?" he asks.

"Yeah," you say. "Good point." You hold up your finger stub. "I guess I can only make small points from now on." You laugh. You like each other. There is no point in trying to re-attach the finger.

"As soon as the operating room is free, we'll take you in there and fix it. We'll have to amputate a little more so we can flap some skin over the bone."

"Is Doctor Lee hogging the OR still?" you ask. It's a lucky guess, but Doctor Luskin seems a bit dumbfounded by it.

"Yes, he is," he says, cocking his head sideways.

"I think I know too many surgeons in this hospital," you say.

He laughs.

Nurses wheel you into the OR after about thirty minutes, mellowed nicely by Doctor Jon D. Schauer with IV sedation. He adds a shot of sedative into the finger itself. The OR seems to be full of people.

Doctor Luskin draws a crowd.

He notes that there is minimal contamination and that the saw blade made an excellent, clean cut. The doctor removes some damaged tissue and then performs a revision amputation, taking away just enough soft tissue and finger structure to create two flaps of skin to pull over the remaining bone.

It creates what is called a fish-mouth type closure, which is sort of what it looks like when a fish closes its mouth.

The doctor removes some nerves, and the bleeding stops.

You are done.

An assistant wheels you up to a room in the hospital. You and Kerstin wait.

A nurse comes in and says they will now admit you.

"I think they want me to go home pretty quick," you say. "I don't think I'm staying here."

"Oh no," she says. "You have to stay here overnight, at least."

"I don't think so," Kerstin says.

Ten minutes later, you are on your way down in the elevator, in a wheelchair that the nurse says you must positively, absolutely sit in, and you go home. Doctor Luskin wants to make sure you don't hang around the hospital, looking for germs.

Your finger heals very quickly. You are playing tennis again two days later. You use your right hand, and the amputation is on the left side. On your service, you learn to toss the ball with three fingers, a big bandage, and a thumb with no problem.

A few weeks later, you are playing doubles with one of your favorite people, Meryl Broadbent. She's a hilarious lady, with an enormous personality, and pretty too. One of your opponents hits a ball beyond the baseline, and you signal it is out with your stubby finger.

"Not as far out as it used to be," she says. You laugh. You have become a master of short finger jokes.

"It took me decades to figure out how to count to ten," you say. "Now, I have to learn to count to nine and a half."

During the changeover, you tell everyone the good news about losing your finger. It has healed very quickly, with no infection and no pain.

Your immune system is chugging away, full throttle. Meryl wants to hold the finger so she can get used to it.

You tell everyone you think you have finally completed your journey from medical dope to healthy hope. The amputation is the journey's final punctuation, an unfortunate exclamation point.

"You know what the good news really is?" Meryl says, letting go of your finger.

"What?" you ask.

"Now, if you hit a great shot, we can give you a high four."

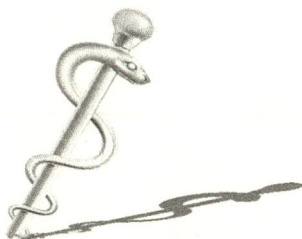

Warrior Patient Rule 17: Laughter relieves stress, boosts immune systems, releases feel-good chemicals in your body, dissolves conflicts, prevents heart disease, and turns threats into a joke. Humor is the best doctor you will ever know.

Chapter 18

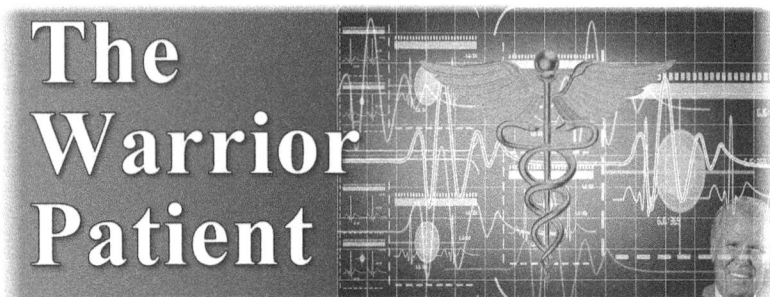

The
Warrior
Patient

We all exist in an extraordinary factory called the human body. While it is working, while it carries us from laughter to tears, the factory is genuinely, magnificently resilient.

This year's model is far superior to the ones available a century ago.

The men and women of medicine continue to improve and prolong all of our fixtures and fittings; they keep moving our expiration date further into the future.

We need to know what to expect from them, what to demand from them.

We need to understand the tools that they use and the mistakes that they make. We need to help them make us better, make our lives better, and longer.

Believe in doctors. Believe in modern medicine. Both can save your life. Know also that you can save your own life, and that is a crucial part of a Warrior Patient's creed. Doctors cannot do it alone. They need a patient willing to fight for his or her life.

Waiting for Doctor Harold Richter, the hematologist (blood specialist), you see some works of art propped up on portable easels in the waiting area. Cancer patients, or someone close to them, create the paintings. Words written beneath each illustration tell the story of the artist who creates it.

The first, a pastel, shows a man with a pitchfork, his back turned, looking across harvested fields into a forest. A sunset of reds, yellows, and blues smothers a distant mountain. The end of another day tinges gray clouds pink. Below the picture is a poem that starts with explosions and red flashes and a tank sprayer spewing Agent Orange in Vietnam. Then 20 years pass. Suddenly, unexpectedly, the artist's prostate trips over a rapidly climbing PSA count. You have been there. You connect. A radical prostatectomy takes him into remission for six years, but his PSA rises again. He fights it with radiation treatments over three dozen times. Three dozen doses of fire bury growing cancer for another seven years. And then it comes back again, and he fights it with his belief in the power of his art and color, symbols of hope and beauty waiting after death. It is another Warrior Patient, humble in his victories.

The next is a photorealistic mixed media by a young woman who has just escaped from her teenage years. She is a lymphoma, mixed cell, stage IVB cancer survivor. Her work of art shows the uplifted face of developing womanhood growing into an uncertain future, but a future bright with colors and patterns. Diseases attack her organs and bone marrow. The oncologists (cancer doctors) give her a 10-20% shot at survival if she makes it through all her treatments. She has a newborn child. She researches her healing process, studies the survival stories of cancer patients, diet, nutrition, spirituality. After her fourth cycle of treatment, she is in remission. She is a Warrior Patient, a survivor, humble in her battle.

The third work of art, almost primitive in its style, shows a leafless tree with its roots cross-sectioned, reaching into the reddish-yellow soil. The background moves from sunrise on the right to blue sky in the middle, and finally to the darkness of night on the left. A small sapling with two green leaves bravely rises beneath the leafless tree.

The artist is the sixteen-year-old son of a cancer survivor who has been given only three months to live.

But his mother is a Warrior Patient, and she fights for her life, and she continues to live beyond the expectations of her doctors.

And her son, the artist, embraces her battle, joins it as the small sapling beneath her tree skeleton, and he will grow, and they will fight as Warrior Patients together, humble in their crusade.

You study these three paintings, and a nurse opens a door and calls your name. The time has come to have your blood drawn and analyzed by the hematologist.

It has been a long journey. For the first time in almost three years, the blood work is perfect. There is no infection. Back to normal. Older. Wiser.

"I'm going to write Doctor Lazar a note saying that you only have to see me if you have a problem," Doctor Richter says.

"I only see Doctor Eric every two or three months now."

There has been no need for dialysis for well over a year. Creatinine levels remain below 2.0. It will always be higher than average, but the kidneys continue to function well. The journey from medical dope to healthy hope is now over.

You stand and shake Doctor Richter's hand, using the extraordinary line that the infectious diseases specialist, Doctor Heiman, used on your final visit to his office. It's a good line, and Doctor Richter laughs well at it.

"I never want to see you again," you say.

When you get back home, Kerstin smiles at "perfect blood."

On television in the living room, they are talking about aging. The subject is pharmaceutical treatments currently available for men with low testosterone levels, Low-T. They discuss the side effects of pill-popping your testosterone count back to a healthy level. The women on the show are laughing, playful. The men are also goofing around, but more intent.

A handsome 41-year-old talking head says: "I will borrow from tomorrow to live for today." People on the show nod with appreciation at this man's sound bite.

It is a terrific line for a guinea pig.

The bean counters watching profit margins in pharmaceutical companies and medical facilities all over America love this kind of guy. He has put his health on a war footing. "Eat, drink and be merry," he suggests, "for tomorrow we die."

The medicine men smile.

Their cash register speaks: "Ka-ching."

It is easy to be stupid in an age of miracles. Anyone born in the 1940s or 1950s knows people who stole cigarettes from their parents and smoked them in secret. When someone suggested to you that they were cancer sticks, you laughed.

"In another twenty years," you said, "they'll have a cure for cancer. We don't have to worry about it."

That was over half a century ago. Of course, surgeons have found a cure. But lung transplants are very expensive, difficult to get, and the entire process remains horrifying, unpleasant, and painful.

The journey of a Warrior Patient from medical dope to healthy hope has many variations, routes, illnesses, soldiers. It raises many questions, some quite disturbing.

Why does a urologist, treating a patient with an apparent infection, ask, "I wonder why you're so infected?" but do nothing about it? And why does his office treat you with abuse instead of kindness when you experience enormous pain?

How does a primary physician prescribe a pain medication that the manufacturer warns might have dangerous consequences if given to a patient suffering from an illness for which the primary physician already treats the patient?

How can a hospital send kidneys into a tailspin after an ultrasound exam shows that they are healthy, leading to kidney dialysis in less than two weeks?

How can a hospital discharge a patient who suffers from renal failure without telling the patient about it, and without indicating the need for kidney dialysis to the patient?

You ask family and friends: "Did all of this have to happen? Was this necessary?"

One answer comes from Filippa Leijonhufvud Reading, a Swedish friend, and fellow Warrior Patient battling cancer with honesty, strength, fear, curiosity, laughter, and tears. She calls herself "The Healing Warrior." She confronts her illness with Body, Mind, and Soul. She tells you that there is a "Godly plan":

"You, Temple, were 'the chosen one' to go through this," she writes. "This comes from a higher power — you, with your healthy, strong body, writing skills, and a good scoop of humor. You were picked to go through this, to document this. FOR A REASON. What you have gone through is important to so many people. Could this have been avoided, changed, re-arranged? I believe not! No! Nope! No way! It's your life path."

Filippa Reading also asks a troubling question: "I am AMAZED that all these Doctors did not connect the dots. Sorry if this might be blunt, but is it that when you're over 70 years of age, they don't care as much? Do younger people get better treatment? More attention? Better service? You're 'over the hill' and might not survive, so why bother?"

Another good friend Michael J. Thomas, an author, writes: "Temple has seen fit to share the experience of a lifetime in hopes that others might benefit. I did, and I think others will. Not that I or anyone else will experience what Temple did, Heaven forbid! But what I got from the book was a sense of salvation through hard work, faith, due diligence, love, respect, and the Grace of God. That makes sense to me."

Many years ago, a Marine Corps demolition instructor explained the profound mystery of survival to me when he said: "The hardest thing in life is to know which bridge to cross and which one to blow up."

The journey from medical dope to healthy hope crosses many bridges, all of them wired for fireworks. But there is common ground and common-sense rules in all Warrior Patient battles. You have seventeen of them (in the chapter order in which they appear).

Chapter 1: Choose to live. Take personal responsibility for getting better. It is not your doctor's job. It is not God's job. It is your job. God and your doctors might help. And they might not.

Chapter 2: The internet unlocks everything you need to know about doctors, hospitals, procedures, and treatments. A mouse, a click, or finger swipe will put you on the right road to solving your medical problems

Chapter 3: Do not accept medical abuse from nurses or technicians. Doctors must eliminate any barriers to good health and human kindness

in their offices, a clinic, a hospital, or any medical facility. Always.

Chapter 4: People usually think their doctor is the best in the world, even if their doctor is in the process of burying them. Trust but verify, also outstanding doctors. Your life will depend on it.

Chapter 5: Cut down on bad habits. Don't smoke, even if you're on fire. Ditch drinking (one glass of wine a day, but no more). Your balance gets much better, in every respect.

Chapter 6: If you need help, get it. Bravery is for dead people. Pain can be a good thing, a roadmap for doctors, but remember that pain pills hide problems, they do not fix them.

Chapter 7: Doctors who go to excellent medical schools are better than doctors who go to poorly-rated medical schools. There are no exceptions to this, NONE.

Chapter 8: Try to understand any tests and procedures your doctors suggest. Many just pay for new hospital equipment. Even good doctors enjoy playing with expensive toys. They get paid well for doing it, too.

Chapter 9: Some physicians like to take a "mushroom" approach to their patients, believing that if they keep them in the dark, they will flourish. Smart patients live longer than dumb ones. *Good* doctors appreciate this fact.

Chapter 10: When you sink into the quicksand of modern medicine, the only way out will be good doctors. Does this violate Rule 1? Not if you're up to your neck in medical quicksand. Grab the rope. Pull hard.

Chapter 11: Death makes people edgy, and healthy folks do not like ill people. So plan your "sick" conversations very carefully. And make sure there's a "for better or worse" clause in your marriage vows.

Chapter 12: Exercise and proper diet are essential medicines. If you screw up on food, start again. If you think you cannot do anything physical, wiggle your toes.

Chapter 13: Do not let today turn into tomorrow's "too late." Get

your shingles shot. Get a flu shot.
Do not die waiting "just one more
day" to visit the doctor.

Chapter 14: Save your medical records. Hospitals can give you a CD of
your info for a few bucks. You may
not understand it all, but it's terrific
reading if you have a hard time
sleeping.

Chapter 15: When a medical facility
asks you for your list of medications, add a list of all your doctors
and medical procedures as well. If
they say they don't need them, consider treatment elsewhere.

Chapter 16: Make sure all your
doctors understand that their reputations depend on how their staff
and office operate, and not just on
how they operate.

Chapter 17: Laughter relieves
stress, boosts immune systems, releases feel-good chemicals in your
body, dissolves conflicts, prevents
heart disease, and turns threats into
a joke. Humor is the best doctor you
will ever know.

Other Warrior Patients may have different rules and regulations. Filippa Reading suggests one: "From the beginning, my oncologist told me to bring a notebook every time I came to see her. Write down questions and also to write down what she said. You do forget over 80% of what's being said." It is a reasonable regulation for Warrior Patients. Rules work.

You know this from personal experience. The journey has now come to an end after almost three years. Like so many other survivors, you have become a Warrior Patient.

Nobody welcomes the next battle, but you know you will fight it well, with toughness, honor, and much more intelligence than you had earlier when your journey began.

Warrior Patients do not win medals.

They win extra sunrises and sunsets, to the end of their days.

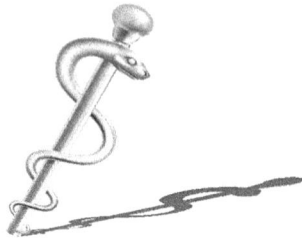

The End

Epilog

In Chapter 7, Doctor Manuel Abreu prescribes pills that you should never take. Your medical history (available on the doctor's computer) contraindicates the medication. The pills help push you into the quicksand of renal failure, kidney dialysis, open wounds, terrible infections, MRSA, partial blindness, shingles, hernias (but not the amputation, that remains your stupidity).

Delray Beach doctor accused of molesting patients

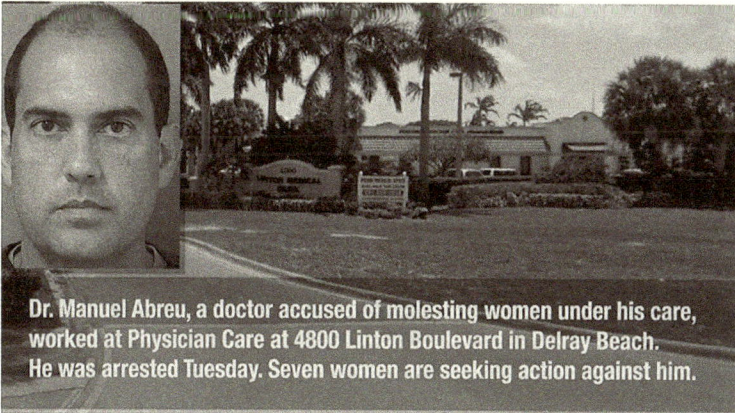

Dr. Manuel Abreu, a doctor accused of molesting women under his care, worked at Physician Care at 4800 Linton Boulevard in Delray Beach. He was arrested Tuesday. Seven women are seeking action against him.

Manuel Abreu is accused of sexual battery.

By Kate Jacobson
Sun Sentinel
contact the reporter

Police arrest Doctor Abreu on March 17, 2015, on criminal charges in Palm Beach County, Florida. They revoke his medical license, and they throw him in jail. The judge sets his bond at half a million dollars.

Seven women lodge additional civil complaints against Doctor Manuel Abreu for violating their trust while in his care. Perhaps that is a fitting end to a graduate of "the 10,623rd best medical school in the world." Friends ask: "Why don't you sue him?"

Your answer: "Who likes standing in a long line?" More important, it would be a shame to have the legal system slap a "gag" order on "Warrior Patient." People need to read it

A quick update on the author's health

Now we are in the age of Covid-19. Before it is over, probably hundreds of thousands of people will die. Kerstin and I are self-quarantined, and we will remain so. It is a great time to be a writer, which, by its nature, includes solitude. We are both in good health, and still in love as well as alive. God bless all of you.

Acknowledgments

Writing has been called a lonely business. It is not. From the start, Warrior Patient overflowed with helpful advice from people, family, and friends. It would take an entire chapter to thank them all. Of course, I would forget someone, and they would not talk to me for a while. It would take weeks to make them laugh about it. They might eventually forgive me. Why run the risk? Time to use the "lump" rule, where you take a bunch of people and bow to all of them in universal, heartfelt gratitude.

To all my friends at the Boca Resort and the Boca Country Club, thank you. So many of you gave me good advice as the book developed. So many of you made the book better, and a few of you even sneaked into its pages. Very few of you talked about me in the past tense, although moments came when it seemed pretty close. You are all spectacular human beings, and some of you are my fellow Warrior Patients. Thank you for your support and for reading my books.

To my family scattered across the face of the globe, thank you. Some of you did not realize how serious my problems became, but I always felt your love and your concern as you went about your busy lives. We are an eclectic bunch, all part of the wondrous Emmet Clan from Ireland, and we protect each other with a tough, creative love that flickers through the ages. Google Robert Emmet. He remains our bedrock, our leader, our giant.

One friend (and her husband) deserve a special nod. Judy Greenman, my proofreader, possesses the eyes of an eagle and the heart of a dove. And I cannot forget her bagman, Brian.

To all the doctors who helped me live, but especially Doctors Donald Heiman and Jose Yeguez. And the most critical medical person of all: Doctor Eric Lazar, who built the path that led me to healthy hope. Thank you. Thank you. Thank you all.

To Brad Hildt, who came from Boston one weekend to make me laugh. He never appeared in the book, but he was always there. "Asante rafiki yangu." Thank you, old friend.

We share a Swahili past.

And finally to the most critical person in my life, my real soulmate for well over 48 years, Kerstin "Kickan" Williams. This book has been described as a self-help memoir, but it is also a romance, a love story to my wife. She has saved my life in so many ways.

Puss och kram. Jag älskar dig varje dag i mitt liv. Kiss and hug. I love you every day of my life.

We share a Swedish Future.

Temple Emmet Williams
2020, and beyond

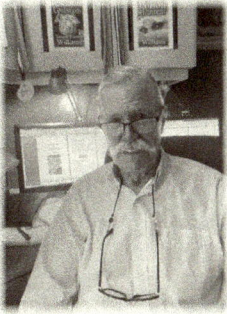

About the Author
Temple Emmet
Williams

Tootie Wright, a childhood neighbor in the small village of Gates Mills, Ohio, where I grew up, sees me dragging a colossal snapping turtle across her lawn in the sweltering heat of July 1951.

"Temple," she calls from her porch, "turn that reptile loose."

Mrs. Wright teaches elementary school with considerable precision. The 15-pound snapper continues its trenchwork across her manicured lawn as I drag it by the tail, upside down, heading straight for —— "Gonna start a turtle farm, Misses Wright."

She bribes me out of the Turtle Business with warm tollhouse cookies. The snapper lumbers back to its nearby pond as Tootie Wright starts reading "The Snow Goose."

Paul Gallico's words paint pictures and run tears down my cookie-crumbed face. Writing fills much of my life after that day as I become a journalist, an editor, a copywriter, a ghostwriter, and a speechwriter. Tootie Wright starts it all.

I also remember the first professional writer who took me under his wing and dared me to make a difference with words: Hayes Jacobs at the New School for Social Research. He wrote in The New Yorker. He would enjoy the significance of the text message near the end of these paragraphs.

Thanks also to all the great newspaper and magazine people who turned me into a journalist, especially Richard D. Peters, my editor at the New York World-Telegram & Sun and Otto Krause at News/Check magazine in South Africa.

Thanks to the incredible editors who turned me into an editor many years later: Ed Thompson and Mary Lou Allin at The Reader's Digest.

Thanks to the great copywriters who taught me the power of words, especially Steve Trygg, David Ogilvy, Leo Burnett, and Rudy Perz (who invented the Pillsbury Doughboy).

My first book, Warrior Patient, had the best review any author could hope for soon after it was published, in a text message on my iPhone:

> **"Going through some medical issues and your experiences have made me look at them in a lighter, better light. It was important for me to let you know your book is helping me deal with and take charge of my treatment. Thanks, Dad."**

Temple Emmet Williams was born in Cleveland, Ohio, and educated at The Hotchkiss School and Yale University.

He became a journalist and was nominated twice for the Pulitzer Prize as an undercover reporter for the World-Telegram & Sun in New York City. He was the Managing Editor of News/Check, an international news magazine in Africa, and an Editor at the Reader's Digest in the United States.

He worked as a copywriter and creative director at large ad agencies around the world, including Ogilvy & Mather and Leo Burnett.

He lived in Africa for six years and in Europe for almost as long. He and his wife, who is his content editor, now live in Boca Raton, Florida, self-quarantined from COVID-19.

"I still have a lot of books to write," says the author.

Please review this book.

How to write a review on Amazon

You have to be a member of Amazon to write a review.

(1) Browse to https://www.amazon.com/dp/B00NRX4WRE

(2) Next to the book's profile picture on the top left, you'll see a "reviews" notice. Tap or click on it.

(3) You'll go to a page that has a box that says: "Write a Customer Review." Tap it.

(4) Write or copy your review into the review box, go through their rating questions, rate it from one to five stars, and save it.

Thank you for spreading the word.

Please read my thrillers.

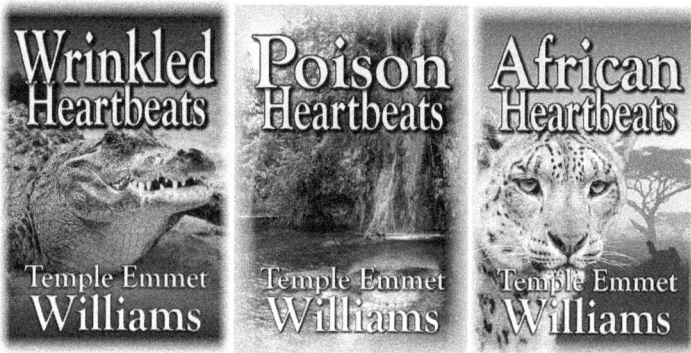

They're all available on Amazon.

www.ingramcontent.com/pod-product-compliance
Lightning Source LLC
Chambersburg PA
CBHW021038090426
42738CB00006B/140